Dangerous and
Disorder

y

This book is to be returned on or before

People with personality disorders are to be found in all branches of psychiatric services, as outpatients, as acute inpatients, and in the community. Their behaviour can be manipulative and threatening and they are hard to manage in institutional settings. *Dangerous and Severe Personality Disorder* is based on a unique research study conducted in the three English High Security Hospitals – Ashworth, Rampton and Broadmoor. Through in-depth analysis of an extensive questionnaire survey followed by personal interviews, Len Bowers shows how positive or negative attitudes to PD patients arise and are maintained over time, discusses what impact these attitudes have upon nurses and the care they provide to patients, and draws some practical conclusions.

The difficulties facing staff who care for and treat PD patients are enormous and constitute a significant personal challenge for the psychiatric professional of any discipline. For the first time this book provides details of the most effective ways of creating a positive context for working with Personality Disorder and offers a blueprint for training and organizational structures across the professional spectrum.

Len Bowers is a psychiatric nurse with a broad experience of inpatient and community psychiatric care. He is Professor of Psychiatric Nursing at the St Bartholomew School of Nursing and Midwifery, City University, London.

Dangerous and Severe Personality Disorder

Response and role of the psychiatric team

Len Bowers

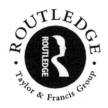

London and New York

First published 2002
by Routledge
11 New Fetter Lane, London EC4P 4EE

Simultaneously published in the USA and Canada
by Routledge
29 West 35th Street, New York, NY 10001

Routledge is an imprint of the Taylor & Francis Group

© 2002 Len Bowers

Typeset in Times by BC Typesetting, Bristol
Printed and bound in Great Britain by
TJ International Ltd, Padstow, Cornwall

British Library Cataloguing in Publication Data
A catalogue record for this book is available from the British Library

Library of Congress Cataloging in Publication Data
A catalog record for this book has been requested

ISBN 0–415–28237–3 (hbk)
ISBN 0–415–28238–1 (pbk)

To Jessica, Sam and George

Contents

Acknowledgements

First thanks go to the two research assistants who worked with me on this project, Linda McFarland and Frank Kiyimba. Their cheerfulness, skill, perseverance and enthusiasm were essential to the final result. Their ideas and thoughts have become so mixed with the development of my own on this topic that they should receive some credit for the contents of this book. As should the rest of my research team, past and present, who have discussed the issues with me, challenged my thinking when necessary, and encouraged me to overcome various obstacles or apparent dead ends. They are: Jane Alexander, Patrick Callaghan, Paola Carr-Walker, Nicola Clark, Neil Crowhurst, Sarah Eales, Catherine Evers (who also carried out the inter-rater reliability exercise), Stuart Guy, Manuela Jarrett, Eddie McCann, Carl Ryan and Alan Simpson. My partner, Eleanor Marshall, was also important in extending my ideas, as well as in giving me consistent and steadfast support throughout the years this work went on. Much support and detailed advice, for which I am most grateful, was also received from my father-in-law, Professor Peter Marshall.

Many others with whom I also discussed the work and exchanged ideas are also deserving of my gratitude, especially Hillary Bradshaw and Jo Paton, and the Steering Group of the research: James Hampton, David Ndegwa, Victoria Hyams, Tony Thompson, Leeanne McGee, David Robinson, Lezli Boswell, Kevin Barron. Christine Hogg of Salford University was helpful in extending my thinking about self-mutilation, Morgan McFarland provided invaluable advice and many superb examples of writing skill, and Lynne Holmes gave me much support during a difficult phase of the data analysis. My thinking was also further developed by the many nurses who asked questions and gave feedback at conference presentations of the findings, within and outside of the High Security Hospitals.

Support from each of the three English High Security Hospitals was enormous. Each devoted time and considerable resources into providing site visits for the induction of the research team. The opportunity for the research team to meet senior staff and nurses on the wards has been absolutely invaluable. Everywhere my team of researchers and I went, we were met with openness and interest. All three hospitals appointed liaison staff to the project, namely

Tony Hopkins, Martin Coupland and Peter Melia. They devoted time to ensuring that the research assistants could access staff for interviews at appropriate times and places. In addition, POA and RCN representatives at the Hospitals gave the project their backing and endorsement. Without this level of support, carrying out the research would have been much more difficult, if not impossible.

The research was funded by the National Programme for Forensic Mental Health Research and Development, who were at every stage supportive and helpful in the execution and reporting of the research. Dilys Jones of the Department of Health was especially encouraging and helpful.

Lastly, but most importantly, I have the highest regard for the psychiatric nurses who work in the High Security Psychiatric Hospitals. In caring for people who have committed serious crimes, they embody and express some of the highest values of our civilisation and culture. The work they do is atrociously difficult, demanding and psychologically pressurised. I have the deepest respect for all of them, even those that fail in their task. They do not receive one-tenth of the public respect and sympathy they deserve. In many ways what I have to present in this book is a summary of their wisdom, experience and knowledge. Without their support and cooperation, there would have been no book at all. The work is therefore largely theirs, and I hope that they feel that I have gone some way towards explaining what it is really like to do the work they do.

1 'Welcome to the world of PD'

'Welcome to the world of PD.' This greeting, offered by one of the nurses I interviewed in an English High Security Psychiatric Hospital, speaks volumes about the chasm that lies between our own everyday lives and that of people suffering from a personality disorder (PD). In that world, actions do not necessarily have the same meaning and consequences, even when they appear to do so. PD patients look the same, talk the same, and in many if not most situations act the same. Yet regularly and periodically they act in ways that demonstrate that they inhabit an entirely different psychological and social world, one where our normal rules for understanding and morally judging behaviour simply do not count. Unlike those who suffer from psychoses, they largely do not have strange beliefs, nor do they hallucinate, hear voices or become disorganised and agitated in their thoughts and actions. However, their view of society and of us is just as perverse, and just as different, if not as obviously evident or visible.

Although the High Security Psychiatric Hospitals are surrounded by high walls and intensive security, those who work there are constantly under the microscope of governmental and public scrutiny. The smallest action can result in critical newspaper headlines. Many of the patients incarcerated there have committed such horrendous crimes that their names are notorious, and familiar to everyone who watches television or reads newspapers. Over the past 30 years a series of high-profile public inquiries has been conducted into these settings and, in addition, industrial action has been taken by the Prison Officers Association – a Trade Union to which many of the nurses belong. Psychiatric nurses working in the hospitals have been accused of meting out harsh treatment to patients and of being overly security conscious. In recent years they have also been accused of the opposite – of not being conscious enough of security and being too soft towards the patients. To be a service manager in this setting is to be vulnerable to the accusation, on the occurrence of any untoward event, of having failed. One way or another, many nurses have lost their careers by working there. A host of concealed dangers and traps thus surround those who deliver nursing care in this setting.

This book describes a research study conducted in the three English High Security Hospitals during 1998–1999. At every level of psychiatric services, from the outpatient clinic to the forensic services, PD patients are an acknowledged problem. Their behaviour is difficult, obnoxious, threatening, and they are hard to manage in institutional settings. It is not easy (indeed sometimes impossible) to engage them in psychiatric treatment over a sustained period of time. Even if one is successful, the outcome of treatment is uncertain. When at large in the community they cause problems for others through their antisocial and irresponsible conduct. Their incessant and contradictory demands upon health service resources (e.g. through repetitive suicidal gestures like overdoses) evoke negative reactions from all professions. Some psychiatric staff reject them completely, seeing them as 'psychological vampires' fully responsible for their behaviour, and appropriate cases for punishment rather than treatment. Yet if held in prison, their behaviour remains disordered. Even in that setting they are difficult to manage, and though recognizably mentally disturbed their transfer to psychiatric care is, in most cases, impossible. Generally speaking, they are people no one wants.

There are, nevertheless, psychiatric nurses who manage to maintain a positive attitude to working with PD patients, viewing them as 'misunderstood misfits', even at the level of PD pathology to be found in those detained within the High Security Hospitals. My study set out to discover what was different about those nurses. How did they manage to sustain a positive approach in the face of the challenges presented by these hostile, obstreperous, demanding and challenging patients? In the course of that study a great deal was learned about the ways in which it is possible to view, understand, conceptualize and respond to personality disordered people who have committed serious crimes. This book is about those findings.

However, it is first necessary to provide some background about personality disorder itself, what it is, what might be its causes, what types of treatment are used, etc. This chapter will provide that information, while the second will describe in a little more detail the research that was conducted. Thereafter the book will be a presentation of, and reflection on, the results.

The provision of a 'state of the art' explanation of PD is by no means easy, as this is an area of psychiatry in which there are many hotly contested debates and arguments. Even the term 'personality disorder' itself is not uniformly used, with the same group of patients (or different subgroups of them) sometimes being called psychopaths or sociopaths. Notwithstanding these disputes, the remainder of this chapter seeks to provide a relatively simple and accessible overview of the psychiatry of PD.

The nature of PD

Perhaps the only thing about personality disorder on which every written authority agrees is that nobody comprehensively knows what it is, which makes my task of describing it quite difficult. There are many competing systems available to describe and categorise PD. Some are based on particular theories about its nature and cause – for example, psychologists who follow trait models of personality use statistically determined models, whereas those from a psychoanalytic background use the theoretical apparatus initially defined by Freud. Other classification attempts have been made by seeking cross-disciplinary consensus on schemes for categorizing those who already receive psychiatric help in one form or another. The two largest of these exercises are the *Diagnostic and Statistical Manual of Mental Disorders* (currently in its fourth edition – DSM-IV) produced by the American Psychiatric Association (1995) and the *International Classification of Diseases* (currently in its tenth edition – ICD-10) produced by the World Health Organization (1989). Although these dominate both debate and clinical practice, the schemes for the definition and classification of personality disorder that they contain are not the same. In fact both attract support and attack in equal measure, with occasional traces of fraying psychiatric temper visible in the literature and at conference debates.

Such is the degree of dissension aroused by the diagnosis of PD that it is hard to come any conclusion other than the whole thing is a terrible mess. New trait psychology terms are introduced and overlap with older, psychoanalytically based psychodynamic models. Descriptive words are used which, although the same (e.g. 'borderline'), can refer to quite different collections of attributes when used by different authors from different traditions. To add more complexity, people with other mental disorders, for example schizophrenia, sometimes also suffer from a personality disorder, while the lifestyle of the PD patient generates stress and dysphoria to the extent of precipitating a mood disorder like depression. Many people with a PD use or abuse drugs, or become addicted through reckless experimentation, leading to additional psychiatric and practical problems. Not only that, but the boundary between PD and other mental disorders is fuzzy, in that many of those suffering from PD also suffer, far more commonly than would be expected through chance, from other mental disorders, e.g. phobias, anxiety, mood disorders and schizophrenia. In the latter case the boundary is even more obscure because some PD sufferers seem to slip transiently in and out of a psychotic state, or acquire false beliefs of a delusional intensity. All efforts at categorizing PD tend to have poor reliability when put to the test. Different schemes describe overlapping, but different, populations. Nevertheless, people with PD exist, suffer, definitely cause problems for others, and occasionally commit serious crimes.

A further element of confusion has been added in the UK by the Mental Health legislation in operation (at the time of writing). The legislation allows courts to detain an offender in a psychiatric hospital under the category of 'psychopath'. As such disposal decisions are made by courts only partly on the basis of properly conducted psychiatric assessments, not all of those legally detained as 'psychopaths' actually suffer from that condition but may, instead, have other psychiatric conditions. In this book we are concerned with those who fit the clinical rather than the legal category of psychopath/personality disorder.

Despite this controversy, the DSM-IV and ICD-10 exercises in psychiatric classification offer a good way to enter the topic and at least begin to describe what people with PD are like as people. To aid me in doing so, I shall use the DSM-IV system, solely on the grounds that it is the one that I personally find easier to describe.

People with a personality disorder are different. They differ in the way that they think, feel, relate to others, and contain (or fail to contain) their impulses. These differences are quite specific in form, dissimilar to other mental disorders such as schizophrenia or depression, and are described in more detail below under the different categories of PD. However, on meeting a person with a PD these differences are not immediately apparent. It might be necessary to spend some time with such patients, know them for a while, ask the right questions or have available reports from others, in order to determine that someone has a PD. Nevertheless, depending on the severity of the condition, it will become apparent quite quickly, for PD leads to distress for the sufferers, or more frequently for those around them who find their behaviour difficult to tolerate. People with a PD thus have poor relationships with others, difficulties at work, etc., and can be severely psychologically and socially disabled. Although those around the PD person may readily recognize that he or she has a problem, the individual does not always accept this. The ways in which PD people act are pervasive and stable over time. In other words, they behave in accord with their disorder in all settings (home, work, socially) and at all times (generally speaking, throughout their adult lives), not just when under stress, or when depressed, or when intoxicated. The ten types of PD listed in the DSM-IV are detailed below.

Antisocial

These PD sufferers care little for the rights or needs of others: thus they are exploitative, manipulative and deceitful to their own benefit. They do not respect the law which they may, through violence or fraud, break at will. They may be impulsive, taking sudden major decisions such as changing employment, relationships, or residence, without thinking through the consequences. Their behaviour is irresponsible and uncontrolled, and they engage in high-risk behaviours without concern for themselves or others (e.g. drunk driving, unprotected sex). Because of their reckless behaviour they find it hard to keep a job, and repeatedly default on social responsibilities – for example, childcare, child support, financial debts. After the event they are not remorseful for their acts, but rationalize them or blame others, including the victims of their crimes.

Avoidant

Those with this type of PD are hypersensitive to criticism, subject to feelings of inadequacy, and find social interaction difficult. They avoid activities where they might experience disapproval or rejection by others, and thus have a restricted range of friends and acquaintances. Even with them they may find it difficult to be intimate, as they fear being shamed or laughed at to an excessive degree. Their emotional response even to very minor criticism, or what they perceive as subtle signs of ridicule, is disproportionately large. They believe themselves to be inferior to others, and in order to feel safe and secure may live a restricted, isolated lifestyle.

Borderline

These people endure unstable emotions, a changeable image of themselves, and impulsiveness. In consequence, their relationships are also fragile and changeable, as the borderline individual swings suddenly between an idealized and a devalued picture of the other. They fear rejection, and respond with extreme emotions to the slightest hint that such a rejection is about to occur. They do not appear to know who they are, and may make sudden changes to their sexual orientation, value system, goals in life, ambitions, etc. Prone to reckless and irresponsible behaviour, they may mutilate themselves or make repeated impulsive suicidal gestures. Such behaviour can occur in the presence of extreme unpleasant emotions (e.g. anger, fear, despair), and, when angry, they may have difficulty in self-control, engaging in outbursts of bitterness, sarcasm or verbal abuse.

Dependent

These sufferers from PD have an excessively strong need for the support and encouragement of others, without which they feel unable to function. Even for trivial decisions they feel they need advice and reassurance from others. Thus they depend upon others to take decisions for them, even major life decisions, and remain passive, allowing themselves to be led. Because their need for others is so strong, they have difficulty is disagreeing or arguing with them (even when circumstances justify anger), as they feel that any conflict risks a withdrawal of the support upon which they are so dependent. They will submit to unpleasant tasks, or even violent or sexual abuse, in order to sustain a relationship upon which they are dependent. The loss of a major supportive relationship will precipitate a desperate and haphazard search for a replacement.

Histrionic

These people are characterized by attention-seeking behaviour and the exhibition of strong emotions. They are charming and like to be the centre of attention in any group. In order to achieve this they behave dramatically, talk theatrically, dress outrageously or in an exaggerated fashion, or act in a sexually provocative or seductive manner. They are easily influenced by others, emotionally taking on board opinions that are strongly expressed, rather than being persuaded through rational argument. Relationships therefore tend to be shallow and changeable.

Narcissistic

Sufferers of this type of PD think very highly of themselves, need (and feel they deserve) a great deal of admiration, and lack empathy with others. They exaggerate their own accomplishments and denigrate the activities or contributions of others, while fantasizing about their own successful achievements or other superior qualities. They seek to associate themselves with people who they see as being of high status, and feel entitled to (and expect) special treatment. Although strongly asserted, their sense of self-importance is, at its core, very fragile. Therefore when others fail to accommodate them, or give due praise or privilege, they may become upset and angry. Also, because they pay no attention to the needs of others, they may behave in a hurtful, exploitative or manipulative fashion.

Obsessive-compulsive

Sufferers from this condition strive for perfectionism at the cost of efficiency. They achieve a sense of control over events through careful attention to rules, details and procedures, but get so engrossed in those things that they may be unable to complete the task they are undertaking. They also set high standards for themselves, sometimes so high that the end result is, again, failure to complete the task in hand through constant changes to the final product. They are devoted to work, and have difficulty taking time off and relaxing, and even when they do, any leisure task is turned into something to be worked at and perfected. They may be highly moral people, following a strict and rigid code of conduct, and may be hypercritical of their own mistakes. They may hoard useless objects in order to ensure that nothing is wasted, be miserly with their economic resources, and find it difficult to delegate tasks or work with others.

Paranoid

These people are mistrustful and suspicious of others. Even in the absence of evidence, they suspect that others harbour harmful plans or intentions towards them. To this end they interpret the behaviour of others as hostile even when it is not. The slightest sign that others are not fully trustworthy is taken as an indication that they are never trustworthy. They are unforgiving of mistakes or slights, imaginary or real, and remain angry for long periods. They may fight back against their originators engaging in attacks which, to the victim, may be unexpected because in reality there has been no insult. Because they lack essential trust in others they do not confide, and find it hard to develop sustained intimate relationships. They are also prone to pathological jealousy over the fidelity of their partner, without any real justification.

Schizoid

Sufferers from this condition are loners who have little interest in social interaction. By their own preference they have few or no friends or confidants, and choose solitary activities of a mechanical nature, rather than those that require company or cooperation. They do not seem to get any, or as much, pleasure as normal people from sensory or interpersonal experiences, and have little interest in sex. They care little what others think of them and are generally socially unresponsive or possibly inept, perhaps appearing to be superficial or self-absorbed.

Schizotypal

These people are very uncomfortable in social situations and eccentric in their behaviour. They may see disconnected events in the world, large or small, local or international, as possessing some unusual meaning, specifically for them. They may be superstitious, or feel that they have paranormal powers or can read others' thoughts, and may engage in informal magical rituals in efforts to produce a desired outcome. Their perceptions may be distorted, and their speech content may be vague or difficult to understand. Because of this, others may consider them odd, social interaction is not smooth, and contact with others may breed anxiety. They have few or no friends, and may also be suspicious of others.

Consequences

It can readily be seen that having a personality disorder is not life enhancing. Sufferers may cause difficulties for others or, in extreme cases, commit serious crimes, but they are unable to live full, productive lives. In the main they find it difficult to sustain positive intimate relationships with others, whether those be friends or partners. They find it difficult to work, or are at best restricted to a range of occupational slots that fit their personality. In short, to a greater or lesser degree, their lives are spoiled by their condition, whether or not they are able to recognize this themselves.

The characteristics of PD are, to a certain extent, quite common. Most of us are capable of behaving in a PD manner on some occasions, or in some contexts, or at certain times in our lives. The difference for an ordinary person is that such ways of behaving do not dominate their interpersonal style. Those characteristics are not consistent across settings or over time, nor are they held to the same extent. It is possible, for example, to be more, or less, empathetic with others, or to be somewhere in between. The person with PD, however, is likely to be found at the far end of the continuum, not just with one undesirable characteristic such as lack of empathy, but rather with many, in patterns that fit the typologies in the DSM-IV, as described above.

PDs in the High Security Hospitals

Making a very crude extrapolation from the figures provided in the DSM-IV, it would seem that perhaps about 1 in 20 people suffer from some form of PD that meets diagnostic criteria. Of course, most of these people manage without ever seeking help or making contact with psychiatric services. Of those who do, many will receive some form of treatment or support as outpatients. Far fewer commit any of the serious crimes that make them eligible for care in the High Security Psychiatric Hospitals. Even within the population of High Security Hospital residents, those solely with a PD diagnosis are in a minority, while many more suffer from psychotic disorders.

In addition to those with PD who are resident in High Security psychiatric care, there are a significant number of people meeting criteria for the diagnosis of PD who are in prison following their serious crimes. Together with those in the High Security Hospitals, these people are known as Dangerous and Severely Personality Disordered (DSPD) in the UK. Careful estimates (Home Office and Department of Health 1999) suggest that there are up to 2,400 DSPD people in the UK, 1,400 in the prison system, 400 in the High Security Hospitals, and 300–600 living in the community. In the UK, a new specialist assessment and treatment service for these DSPD individuals is now being piloted. Controversially, there is in addition an intention to pass legislation that will permit preventive detention of those currently living freely in the community.

Serious violence against others was the common denominator of the crimes committed by PD patients detained in the High Security Hospitals. The following information comes from Coid's (1992) survey of PDs in both the High Security Hospitals and prisons in the UK. The crimes leading to their detention included: murder, manslaughter, attempted murder, assaults of various types with and without weapons, robbery, aggravated burglary, kidnap, rape, buggery, indecent assault, arson, fraud, blackmail, etc. The motive for many of these crimes was sadistic violence, involving torture and sexual abuse. Some PDs had killed more than once. Coid gives the example of one man who made two armed attacks on women, 'then after his perceived rejection by his family and a male sexual partner, he shot his 11-year-old sister with an air pistol, beat her to death with a brick, and buggered her' (p. 89). Just under a third of patients admitted to sadistic fantasies of rape, torture or homicide, and many masturbated to these fantasies, or had acted them out in hospital or during their criminal offences. Sexual sadism was not only a feature of male PD patients, it also occurred in female patients. Violence against the person was less frequent among the crimes of female PD patients, but arson was a feature of half the index offences of female patients. Detention in prison or hospital did not necessarily bring to an end the offending career of PDs, some of whom managed to murder, or attempt to murder, fellow inmates. Coid describes how 'one man had persuaded another to fake a hanging attempt in order to be sent to hospital. After placing the noose around the other's neck, he kicked away the chair and tried to hasten his victim's demise by pulling on his legs before prison officers could intervene' (p. 87).

In the same study, Coid compared PD patients detained in the High Security Hospitals with prisoners in three special prison units developed to contain seriously disruptive prisoners. The vast majority (98 per cent) of these prisoners met the criteria for a diagnosis of personality disorder; in fact they met the criteria for a mean of 4.4 PD categories each, indicating that they were more pathological than the High Security Hospital population. A significant proportion of these prisoners had previously resided within the High Security Hospitals, but had been transferred to prison because of their unmanageable behaviour in the hospital setting. These findings indicate that a proportion of prisoners in the UK are clinically indistinguishable from the PD population of the High Security Hospitals, justifying the creation of a new DSPD specific service to deal with both groups together.

Cause of PD

There are many theories, much suggestive information, and few well-supported facts about the cause of PD. Theories range from genetic through neurological to developmental. Each explanation has some empirical support, so it may well be that what we call PD is, in reality, a mixed bag of different conditions caused in different ways, or that PD is a final common end point of different events, or that it takes a combination of different aetiological factors to bring about PD. The literature on the cause of PD is vast, and only a brief overview can be provided here.

The fact that we all possess some PD characteristics to some degree has led trait psychologists to consider that the condition of PD itself merely represents one end of the continuum of normal personality variation. Or, that PD occurs when several of these independently varying characteristics occur, in the extreme, together. This view is perhaps supported by results from the use of measurement scales for PD (checklists of characteristics or questionnaire items used in research to define PD), which demonstrate that the features of PD do seem to vary naturally in extent and degree across any population. Building on this, some psychologists have sought to unify thinking about PD with existing, well-developed and empirically based theories about the differing dimensions of personality like the popular Five Factor Model. Others have sought to develop new theories about the dimensions of personality based on study of PD traits, for example Livesley *et al.* (1992) postulate that the four relevant dimensions of personality are 'emotional dysregulation', 'dissocial behaviour', 'inhibitedness' and 'compulsivity'. A recent overview of these arguments can be found in Parker and Barrett (2000). This has led to explanations of PD based on Darwinian evolutionary thinking, i.e. that PD personality traits have evolved and survived in human populations through natural selection. They confer, in some way, a survival advantage. Others completely reject this picture, arguing that PD is categorically and qualitatively different from normal personality. However, perhaps this is just the sense generated by contact with people at the extreme, who give the disconcerting impression, over time, of being wholly other, living in a world of entirely different relevancies and social perceptions.

If PD were the extreme end of variation in personality type, as trait psychologists think, then it would seem likely that evidence showing a genetic contribution to other personality traits also implies that PD is to some extent genetically determined. Plomin *et al.* (1997) argue that there is evidence, much of it from studies of twins, demonstrating that nearly half of all differences in personality traits are accounted for by inheritance. By extrapolation, this may also hold for PD. There is also evidence that PD 'runs in families', suggesting that genetic inheritance may be a component of the cause. For example, relatives of people with Borderline PD are five times more likely than the general population to suffer from this form of PD. It is also associated with an increased risk of Antisocial PD, which is itself more frequent among first-degree relatives than would be expected by chance. However, genetic inheritance is not the whole story, as both adopted and biological children of parents with Antisocial PD have a greater risk of developing the disorder themselves (Cloninger and Svrakic 2000). These facts have led to complex theories about the way genetic inheritance of personality traits interacts with early environment and experience (Millon and Davis 1996).

The view that PD is some form of physiological brain disorder finds some support from many different strands of evidence. Physiological disorder may not necessarily be an inherited condition, but may instead be due to brain damage acquired through, for example, birth trauma. Electroencephalograph (EEG) studies of people with PD, especially those who are violent and aggressive, tend to show abnormalities associated with immature brain development. In addition, there have been several studies that assessed the neurological functioning of people exhibiting antisocial behaviour (e.g. juvenile offenders, psychopaths, forensic psychiatric inpatients) which have shown minor neurological signs of developmental disabilities in neuropsychological tests. For example, Sellars (1992) found that half of his sample of PD patients in a UK High Security Psychiatric Hospital suffered from neurological impairment. Finally, there appears to be some form of link between PD and attention deficit hyperactivity disorder (ADHD), as follow-up studies of hyperactive children have shown that some grow up to have a personality disorder. ADHD itself is associated with minimal brain dysfunction and is thought to be, in part, an inherited condition.

Other causal accounts of PD look to the childhood upbringing and experience of sufferers as playing a major role. The largest body of hard empirical evidence on this comes from long-term longitudinal studies of antisocial behaviour and the family background of those who display such behaviour. Such studies incorporate significant numbers suffering from a PD, especially Antisocial PD. Other causal explanations, based on childhood development, are derived from studies of the psychology of PD sufferers themselves, together with longstanding theoretical traditions in psychiatry (namely psychoanalytic, and cognitive-behavioural).

Taking the longitudinal studies first, West and Farrington (e.g. Farrington 1991) have followed up for nearly thirty years a sample of over 400 8-year-old London boys from a working-class background. By the age of 25, one-third had acquired a criminal conviction of some sort. Three subgroups of offenders could be identified: those with a single juvenile offence; temporary recidivists who had multiple convictions during youth but stopped on reaching adulthood; and persisting delinquents who continued to offend. The last group overlaps with Antisocial PD, and adverse features identified by age 10 which distinguished them from others were:

- very poor parental behaviour, e.g. conflict, dominance, inconsistency, indifference, rejection, neglect, erratic or harsh discipline;
- very large family size;
- both parents convicted of offences;
- low income family.

These findings reflect other, similar studies. For example, Robins (1966) followed up children who had been referred to a child guidance clinic for antisocial behaviour. As well as discovering that many grew up to continue their antisocial behaviour, Robins also found that many came from backgrounds of parental alcoholism, conflict, desertion and neglect. These studies strongly suggest that these factors during upbringing have a causative role in the development of Antisocial PD.

Cognitive-behavioural accounts of the cause of PD seek to explain the emergence of patterns of thinking, emotional responsiveness and belief. Some of these causal accounts are fairly simplistic, asserted without the provision of empirical evidence, and used only to bolster particular therapeutic strategies. For example, Beck and Freeman (1990) suggest that rejection during childhood causes the development of a negative self-image. Repeated experiences of rejection make the belief structuralized, and the person avoids further repetition of pain by not engaging in situations where it may recur, hence developing the features of Avoidant PD. Other cognitive-behavioural theories are more complex and articulated, such as Linehan's (1993) explanation of the development of Borderline PD. In this case the aetiological theory is explicitly linked to a particular conception of what Borderline PD is: high emotional vulnerability plus an inability to regulate or correctly identify emotions, tolerate distress or trust one's own emotional responses as valid. Linehan finds causal elements of this disorder in emotionally invalidating environments experienced during childhood, the imposition of gender role stereotypes, inherited vulnerabilities and childhood abuse (especially childhood sexual abuse). She is able to marshal a wide range of empirical evidence from psychology on child development, on differences in emotional responsiveness, plus the strong correlation between Borderline PD and childhood abuse, in order to support her case. Nevertheless, in Linehan's writings too, the main focus is on effective treatment for PD rather than exploration of the causal mechanisms by which it occurs, a pragmatic focus that is common to most cognitive-behavioural approaches to PD.

In a similar way, most causal explanations of PD given by psychiatric professionals working in the psychoanalytic tradition also have a three-part focus. They account for the cause of the disorder in a style that formulates in a certain way the essential nature of PD. These accounts are then integrated within a particular treatment approach. In their review, Higgitt and Fonagy (1992) point to three current psychoanalytic theories on the cause of PD. That of Kohut (1977, 1984) is fairly typical, and suggests that a profound fault occurs in the early childhood environment of those who become personality disordered. An excessively unempathic response from parents means that the development of the self is arrested and stuck at a primitive level. During normal development, infants see the parent as part of themselves. Through soothing, caring and consistent nurturance, the parent holds the infant (psychically) together. In the absence of that empathic containment, to support self-cohesion and self-esteem, the infant is forced to use pathological methods such as grandiosity or rage – a process accompanied by much inner emptiness and psychic pain. This frustrated development is carried through into adulthood where it results in the presentation known as PD. Other theories differ in detail about the psychological mechanisms involved, but likewise find the cause of PD in problems with the infant's earliest experiences with caretakers. These theories are derived mainly from observation and reflection upon the responses of patients during psychotherapy, but also from systematic observation of mother–infant interaction.

It is not possible to come to a definitive conclusion about the cause of PD. Unfortunately much of the evidence we have is suggestive rather than definitive. Scientific work has been complicated by the diagnostic confusion of PD and its subtypes and the differing definitions used at various times in different studies make it difficult to compare results. Also, most evidence about aetiology refers primarily to Antisocial or Borderline PD. The cause of other varieties of PD remains relatively uninvestigated. Perhaps the best that can be said at this point is that the cause of the problems of PD patients who reside in High Security Psychiatric Care in the UK is probably multifactorial. This is underlined by Coid's (1992) study, which showed that nearly all his subjects had adverse factors in their background from one or more of the following groups:

- genetic (mentally ill or personality disordered first degree relative);
- neurological (birth trauma, developmental delay, etc.);
- environmental factors during childhood (abuse, loss of parents, domestic violence, poverty, criminality).

Treatment of PD

Virtually everything in the psychiatric armamentarium has been tried on the sufferers of PD at one time or another. In their review, Dolan and Coid (1993) have brought together all current research evidence on the efficacy of various approaches to treatment, and this section of the book draws heavily on their work. It would be very pleasant to be able to report that specific treatment methods were effective or had good outcomes. Unfortunately the picture is not so clear, as will be seen.

Every class of psychotropic medication has been prescribed to PD patients in valiant efforts to improve their condition. However, there are complications in judging whether medication has been helpful or not. As has already been pointed out, many sufferers of PD have additional psychiatric problems. Any improvement consequent to taking medication may thus be due to an alleviation of these conditions, many of which are known to respond well to pharmacological treatment (e.g. depression or schizophrenia). A further problem in judging whether medication ameliorates the condition of PD is the fact that rigorously controlled studies have not yet been carried out. Such randomized controlled trials (RCTs) represent the gold standard in terms of evidence for the efficacy of any therapeutic treatment. People suffering from a known condition (for example, PD) are randomly allocated to experimental or placebo treatment, and their response assessed by staff who do not know the condition to which the individual patients have been subject (thus reducing bias in the results). In fact this type of trial has been rarely carried out with sufferers of PD, and not at all with any pharmacological treatment. What evidence there is appears to suggest that some psychotropic medications may have some utility in the symptomatic treatment of particular personality disorders (e.g. lithium or carbemazepine may reduce aggressive outbursts, antidepressants may have some value in ameliorating Borderline PD). There is no evidence that any medication is an effective treatment for the underlying condition of PD. A further layer of complexity is added by the known tendency of PD people to abuse legitimate and illegitimate drugs. Therefore, even if a psychotropic compound was discovered to have a beneficial impact, it may still be used abusively by PD patients (e.g. minor tranquillizers such as valium, or low-dose amphetamines such as ritalin).

Physical treatments have also been tried, without any definitive success. For example, electroconvulsive therapy (ECT) has been demonstrated not to work. Psychosurgery has also been used in times past as a treatment for PD, but there are no rigorous findings on whether it was helpful in the long term. In any case, such a radical, permanent treatment – which, in addition, carries a high risk of death – cannot really be ethically justified.

Psychodynamic psychotherapy is a tool commonly used in the treatment of PD. At its most intensive, this can require four or more one-to-one meetings with a therapist every week, whereas at the other end of the spectrum it can be conducted on a weekly group basis (i.e. one therapist with several patients meeting for an hour). It is hard to generalize about therapy of this type, as there are so many different styles and theories. Most seek to enhance patients' insight into their own inner emotional life and consequently their behaviour, thus promoting behavioural control and change. In individual therapy, it is the patient's feelings towards the therapist, and the interpretation of those feelings, that provide for the growth in insight. In group-oriented approaches it is the relationship, feelings and behaviours between members of the group, plus the ongoing group process, which provide a comparable experience. Experts in this approach see treatment for many years as the ideal.

Psychotherapy literature acknowledges that PD patients are much more difficult to work with than others because of their intense and fluctuating feelings towards their therapists, plus the negative feelings that they evoke in their therapists. At one moment patients can be extremely demanding and dependent on the therapist whom they see as an omnipotent rescuer; the next, responding with aggression and anger, they regard the therapist as a persecutor who is seeking to destroy them. Patients may disrupt the treatment by missing sessions, coming late (or drunk), threatening violence or suicide, self-harming or self-mutilating just before or just after therapy. The therapists need to contain their own natural reactions to these strong but distorted communications and feelings, assisting the patients to see through them to the reality.

Evidence for the efficacy of psychodynamic psychotherapy is, unfortunately, not conclusive. According to Dolan and Coid (1993), although several studies have shown short-term benefits, others have shown that those benefits disappear over the longer term. The groups on which these studies have been based have been diverse (e.g. some on adolescent delinquents and others on prisoners) and the type of therapy has varied. These aspects of the research that has been carried out undermine any attempt to generalize from their findings. The best that can be said is that psychotherapy may be effective.

Cognitive-behavioural therapy can be viewed as an alternative psycho-therapeutic treatment, but one that arises out of a completely different theoretical tradition. The focus of this type of therapy is to assist patients to change their biased judgements of events and the cognitive errors that go to make up their particular personality disorder. Therapy is thus usually made up of individual sessions where, through dialogue and the analysis of current events in the patient's life (or in the therapeutic encounter itself), the precise details of the patient's thinking and interpersonal interpretative style are uncovered, and alternative explanations and interpretations are explored. Homework tasks may be set for patients to try different ways of responding, complete diaries of events and their own emotional reactions and behaviour for further discussion in therapy, or to test their interpretation of events in personal 'experiments'. In addition, such therapy is sometimes accompanied by group sessions in which patients are taught and experiment with a range of new social skills so that they can manage better in their relationships with others. There are also generic problem-based group therapy approaches employing cognitive-behavioural principles – for example, anger management group programmes which are widely used with PD patients in forensic psychiatric settings.

Specific cognitive-behavioural strategies have been devised for all types of PD (Beck and Freeman 1990), but have not been rigorously evaluated for any except perhaps Borderline PD. The latter is notable for having been evaluated by RCT and shown to reduce self-harming behaviours. Short-term beneficial effects of anger management training have also been demonstrated. Although cognitive-behavioural approaches are relatively new in the treatment of PD, they have been shown to work well with other mental disorders, and even with those suffering from psychosis. There is a great deal of hope that this will be effective in the treatment of PD, but it will take some time for evidence to accumulate as to whether or not this is so.

The behavioural treatments that have been tried are token economies and social skills training, or a combination of both. Token economies are where patients on a ward are rewarded for positive behaviours with tokens which can be exchanged for goods or privileges. They were popular in the 1970s and used widely in the rehabilitation of the chronically mentally ill who had become institutionalized in hospitals. Social skills training is usually carried out on a group basis and involves detailed instruction in the social skills of daily life, e.g. making conversation, striking up acquaintance, verbal assertion, etc., plus role play in the group and homework sessions in between group meetings. Although not specifically tested with PD patients, these behavioural treatments have been tried with a variety of young offenders. The results were encouraging in the short term (e.g. reductions in aggressive behaviour) but tended to fade quickly over the longer term. Token economies are no longer popular, as illustrated by the fact that these evaluative studies all took place in the 1970s (e.g. Cohen and Filipczak 1971). Social skills training continues to be used, or is subsumed in other more comprehensive cognitive-behavioural treatments like Dialectical Behaviour Therapy (DBT) or anger management programmes.

One of the most prominent treatments for PD has been that of the Therapeutic Community (TC). TCs were a UK initiative, initially used during World War II as a treatment for shell-shocked or battle-fatigued servicemen (Main 1946). After the war, that work developed in a number of different directions, with TC principles being applied to the care of all sorts of people with all sorts of problems (e.g. in the old asylums for the mentally ill, in the treatment of alcoholism and drug addiction, in prisons for violent offenders or disruptive prisoners). However, TCs primarily became seen, within psychiatry, as the treatment of choice for PD, as exemplified by two internationally famous TCs specializing in its treatment, the Henderson and the Cassel. Although enormously influential in terms of ideology, these units were small and only available to a very tiny proportion of those suffering from PD in the UK. At the peak of TC popularity, many psychiatric hospitals experimented with either creating TCs or applying TC principles to their current work. However, TC treatment was never widely available, although that situation has been changing over the last few years with the creation of two new offshoots of the Henderson Hospital.

Therapeutic Communities operate according to four principles (Rapoport 1960): democratization, with residents and staff sharing in decision-making; permissiveness, the tolerance of distressing and deviant behaviour; communalism, as exemplified by shared amenities, free communication and use of first names; and reality confrontation through which patients receive continuous feedback on their behaviour as seen by others in the community. Kennard (1998) further describes the features of TCs that embody these values, such as frequent group meetings for the sharing of information, building sense of community cohesion, open discussion and decision-making, provision of feedback to individuals on their behaviour. He goes on to outline how, in TCs, residents are expected to contribute to the maintenance and running of the community (e.g. cooking, cleaning, decorating, etc.). This contribution serves a variety of purposes: it binds people together, enhancing cohesion, provides an opportunity to exercise practical life skills, and embodies and expresses the ideal of social responsibility. Most importantly the interpersonal difficulties of residents will surface and emerge clearly through shared tasks. Those difficulties can then be examined publicly in group meetings, providing opportunity for residents to learn from their difficulties, or be confronted with the effect of them on others. Allied to this idea is the fact that TC residents are not just recipients of therapy, but are involved in the provision of that therapy to other residents. Hence they, too, give feedback and interpret each other's behaviour. Although the process of therapy is seen as one of 'learning', the interpretive schema used by staff is usually that of psychodynamic psychotherapy, because many of the founding fathers of the TC approach were themselves psychotherapists (e.g. Ffoulkes, Bion).

Evaluative studies of TCs have shown good results for patients with PD, although those results are not incontrovertible. Improvements in psychological measures, aggressive behaviour, reductions in distress have been shown in the short term; however, no long-term impact upon offending behaviour has been adequately demonstrated. The application of TC principles in the High Security Hospital environment is problematic, although attempts have been made to introduce the treatment. In a traditional TC, patients reside there voluntarily and although their behaviour is difficult, they do not pose the same serious risk to others as do High Security Hospital residents. Thus when TCs have been tried in the latter setting, they have had to be somewhat modified, as they also have when managing similar residents in prison settings.

The treatment offered to patients with PD in the High Security Hospitals is very variable, and how the organization of treatment for PD is different in each of the three English High Security Hospitals will be described in the following chapter. Even within individual hospitals, the treatment received by individual patients can be inconsistent, and variable over the course of their stay. This has led some to say that treatment for these patients is 'haphazard' (Brett 1992). Dell and Robertson (1988) examined the treatment of 106 psychopaths who had been in Broadmoor for an average of 8 years, and discovered that 71 per cent had been in group therapy, 43 per cent in individual therapy, 42 per cent in other psychological treatment, and 14 per cent were on psychotropic medication at the time of the study. A startling 16 per cent had received no specific treatment during their stay. Perhaps this variation in treatment approaches is not surprising, given the absence of convincing evidence as to which approach is most effective. Without that evidence, treatment is likely to be determined by the sympathies and beliefs of individual psychiatric professionals, disciplinary teams, or managers.

A large number of studies have looked at the generic outcome of treatment within the High Security Hospitals (Dolan and Coid 1993). This research has followed up patients after discharge from hospital, without detailing the content of the treatment they had received. It shows that, as judged by re-offending or recall to hospital, outcome for patients with PD is worse than those detained with other mental illnesses. About half of all PD patients commit a further crime within three years. In half of these reoffences, the crime is serious or violent. How these figures are interpreted is, like beauty, in the eye of the beholder. They can be viewed as demonstrating a 75 per cent success rate for hospital treatment, or a 50 per cent failure rate.

Attitudes of psychiatric professionals to PD

It is almost a truism to state that psychiatric nurses (and psychiatrists, Lewis and Appleby 1988) tend to dislike personality disordered patients. Moran and Mason (1996: 189) write of personality disorder within the High Security

Hospitals, that 'Few psychiatric nurses prefer to care for this patient group and tend to dislike this population.'

In the psychiatric literature, a link between difficulties in inpatient management and subsequent suicide has been made, mostly in relation to those patients considered to be suffering from Borderline Personality Disorder (BPD). Adler (1973), Friedman (1969) and Gunderson (1984) all describe increasing malfunctioning and suicidal behaviour of patients within the context of negative reactions by staff, in a form very similar to that which Morgan and Priest have termed malignant alienation. Kullgren (1985), in a retrospective analysis of 11 cases of BPD who committed suicide during inpatient treatment, showed that in more than half the cases rejecting or repressive characteristics could be found in the treatment given. Using a similar methodology, but adding a matched control group of BPD sufferers who did not commit suicide, Kullgren (1988) showed that for 5 of 11 completed suicides, discharge was being planned due to perceptions that the patients were manipulative, or that they were not suffering from serious psychiatric disorder.

Many mental health professionals feel particularly alienated from patients diagnosed as having a BPD (Gallop *et al.* 1989). Although there is considerable controversy about the nosologicial status of this disorder, most mental health professionals agree that the term is useful (Spitzer *et al.* 1979). Such patients are likely to harm themselves repeatedly (Brodsky *et al.* 1995) and commonly induce strong countertransference reactions in staff (Rosenbluth 1991).

Two reviews of the nursing literature (May and Kelly 1982, Ganong *et al.* 1987) on 'good' and 'bad' patients show that nurses tend to express negative judgements about patients who are perceived as (a) hostile, uncooperative, complaining and manipulative; (b) suffering from chronic or stigmatized illnesses; (c) making staff feel ineffective. Personality disordered patients fit several of these characteristics, and studies of nurses show that they also have negative responses to patients who self-harm (e.g. Sidley and Renton 1996, Suokas and Lonnqvist 1989).

Plentiful evidence exists that nurses become alienated from disliked patients. Using systematic observation techniques, Hamera and O'Connell (1981) demonstrated reduced numbers and duration of contacts with such patients, as did a study by Podrasky and Sexton (1988). An alternative approach to investigating this issue has been in-depth qualitative interviews with nurses. Using this methodology, Smith and Hart (1994) showed that intense encounters with angry patients could lead to nurses disconnecting and withdrawing from patients, and McCrea and Crute (1991) found that midwives reported avoiding patients who, in their eyes' 'had no clear needs'. Also, MacIlwaine (1981) reported that, on acute psychiatric wards, neurotic patients are viewed by nurses as 'not really ill', and tend to be ignored. The concept of malignant alienation was first introduced by Morgan and Priest (1984) and was based upon their analysis of 26 unexpected deaths among psychiatric inpatients. They discovered that a significant number of patients who committed suicide lost support from others in the last few weeks of their lives. Staff became critical of the behaviour of these patients, which was perceived to be provocative, unreasonable and over-dependent. Morgan and Priest termed this process 'malignant alienation'. They later replicated these findings (Morgan and Priest 1991), showing that out of a further 32 completed suicides of psychiatric inpatients, 15 had become alienated in some degree from others. Although Watts and Morgan (1994) discussed the phenomenon from a psychodynamic perspective, no further empirical work has been carried out.

Summary

Surprisingly little is concretely known (or agreed) about people with PD, despite the fact that they cause serious problems for any community or society. They behave in ways that are disruptive of personal relationships, family life, employment and leisure activity, and they do this both consistently and persistently. They do the same with those people who try to help them in psychiatric clinics and wards. At the more serious end of the scale they may commit serious crimes that lead to their long-term detention in a forensic psychiatric institution or prison. They are psychologically and socially disabled by the ways in which they behave towards others, and are prevented from leading a fulfilling life. They see the world, society, themselves and other people in a very distorted fashion. Large numbers of people, perhaps as many as 1 in 20 of the population, suffer from these disorders to some degree. Yet the attitude of psychiatric professionals towards them, is, in general, profoundly negative. Many believe them to be either untreatable (and therefore should be ignored by psychiatric services), or not to suffer from a mental disorder at all (being bad rather than mad). These negative attitudes are accentuated by the difficult, disruptive and rejecting behaviours of PD sufferers. Even within the High Security Psychiatric Hospitals, they are not a popular patient group to work with.

Years of debate and of careful descriptive work have not resulted in a single widely accepted system of classification for these disorders – a fact that has severely handicapped research on their cause, treatment and outcome. Although the causes are known to be part genetic, part neurological damage, and part early childhood deprivation or abuse, little is known specifically about the relative contribution of these different factors in individual cases. Many different treatment approaches have been tried, and although some are promising, we still lack firm evidence that any of them work effectively, but it would also be true to say that we do not have evidence that comprehensively establishes that they do not work. However, therapeutic pessimism about PD is widespread among psychiatric professionals, adding to negative attitudes towards PD patients who are, in any case, not easy to engage in any treatment.

2 'Special Hospital country'

Life within the High Security Hospitals (previously called the Special Hospitals, or just 'the specials' – large institutions with a chequered history, populated by patients like the personality disordered who in an everyday sense appear to be normal, although their behaviour is not – can only appear strange to the outsider. It is so radically different from everyday life that one interviewee referred to it as 'Special Hospital country', in other words a land of different customs, traditions, language and values. The sense of difference is exacerbated by the high walls, the ritual security measures and searches on entry, and the profound moral implications of the residents' previous crimes.

This chapter will introduce the research on which this book is based and describe its methods and preliminary findings. However, in order to understand what nurses have to say about caring for PD patients in these environments, it is also necessary to know something about the history of the institutions within which that care takes place, and the way in which it is organized.

The organization of PD care

Until the 1990s, patients with PD were spread throughout the High Security Hospitals with small numbers on any one ward. As they were such a demanding type of patient, it was considered that keeping them and predominantly psychotic patients together actually aided in their management. However, this prevented the development of specialist treatment and the gathering together of specialist professional expertise in the management of PD patients. Therefore recent years have seen the development of PD units in each of the three High Security Hospitals.

Late in 1993, as part of the response to the Blom-Cooper Report (Blom-Cooper et al. 1992) – see below – Ashworth Hospital reorganized and opened a special unit for patients with PD. This was composed of six wards catering for 130 patients, and is said by Storey et al. (1997) to be the largest single unit of its type in Europe. Nurses were allocated to work on this unit regardless of their wishes and desires. As this was the first such unit in High Security Hospitals, the staff had little specific experience upon which to draw, and the necessity for training input was identified at an early stage. Given the paucity of literature on the practical psychiatric nursing care of this difficult group of patients, staff had to create a regime and culture by themselves. The downside of this situation has been the number of untoward events resulting in internal and external inquiries. Among the benefits has been the development, by trial and error, of psychiatric nursing expertise in dealing with the personality disordered individual. This is now being shared, via the literature, by nursing staff from Ashworth Hospital (e.g. Melia *et al.* 1999, Moran and Mason 1996).

The PD unit at Rampton Hospital is of fairly recent origin, being founded as a single ward in 1996 and is now a three-ward unit consisting of admission, treatment and pre-discharge wards. Although planned within a remarkably short time-scale (8 weeks), the unit has followed a policy of only recruiting staff who actively apply to work there (in contrast to Ashworth). The unit has defined admission criteria, prefers to take transfers of sentenced prisoners, and the primary diagnoses of most patients are Antisocial and/or Borderline Personality Disorder. Treatment is mainly cognitive-behavioural in emphasis, although some therapeutic community principles are followed.

Unlike the other two hospitals, Broadmoor does not have a personality disorder unit with its own separate identity. However, it does have several wards where patients with personality disorder tend to be concentrated. The first is Glastonbury ward, an addictive behaviours unit using a very broad definition of addiction and well described by McKeown *et al.* (1996a, 1996b). The second is Woodstock ward, which specializes in the care of young male patients (Brett 1992). The third is Leeds, a female ward where the dominant diagnosis is that of personality disorder. These three wards have been in operation for some years in accord with their current philosophy.

Although this may give the impression that care for PD is neatly and comprehensively organized within the High Security Hospitals, things are not quite as tidy as they appear. Senior clinicians in each hospital operate different diagnostic criteria for PD and therefore for entry to the PD units. In addition, different patient flows at different times have meant that different types of patients have accumulated on the different units, with a large number of high-profile patients at Ashworth Hospital who are unlikely to be discharged and who therefore have less motivation to engage in treatment. Within all three of the hospitals, there are many patients with PD who still reside on wards which contain a majority of psychotic patients. This is particularly likely where the patients suffer from both personality and psychotic disorder. Lastly, as can be seen from the descriptions above, units at the different hospitals offer different treatments and operate according to different philosophies.

The inquiry culture

Psychiatry as an institution has always been controversial, subject in the past 300 years to a number of scandals and inquiries (Jones 1972). More recently in the UK, in the 1960s, 1970s and 1980s, the psychiatric care provided in institutions came under sustained criticism for poor standards, abuses of care and neglect of patients. Martin (1984) details a sequence of highly public inquiries, which were reported widely in the UK national press, into the care provided in these institutions. This public disillusionment with institutional, asylum-based care, provided part of the energy behind the move to community care for the mentally ill in the UK – a move that has resulted in the closure of many of the old asylums dating back to the mid-nineteenth century, and the opening of smaller psychiatric units, typically situated in general hospitals, providing short-term inpatient care only. Not that this has brought to an end the inquiries and scandals that have consistently dogged the practice of psychiatry. Instead the criticism has moved to the practice of mental health professionals in the community, and a yet greater number of public inquiries, typically following homicides perpetrated by the mentally ill (Sheppard 1996).

Perhaps, not surprisingly, forensic psychiatric care has also been subject to a similar process. However, the intensity and public scrutiny associated with that process has been, arguably, greater than that directed at general psychiatry. Probably this is because some of the patients residing in the High Security Hospitals are notorious, nationally known figures that attract strong negative affect from the public. Anything that involves them is therefore considered newsworthy by the Press, and provides an opportunity to repeat descriptions of the horrifying crimes they have committed. Furthermore, since the High Security Hospitals are less open to public scrutiny because of necessary security measures, hence there is a continuous sense of suspicion about what happens behind the walls, within the security perimeter. Lastly, recidivism by those discharged is newsworthy, and readily made to appear as failure on the part of the professionals who work within these institutions.

It is not possible to describe in detail all the inquiry reports that have been written about High Security Hospital care. However, as they provide a major context to current clinical practice, and especially current government policy towards serious offenders who are personality disordered, an overview is required in order to make better sense of some of the research findings.

In 1979 a television documentary alleged that patients in Rampton Hospital were ill treated by staff, and these allegations led not only to police investigation, but also to the setting up of a public inquiry to review the care provided at Rampton. At this time there were no specialist PD units within the High Security Hospital system, and PD patients were cared for on wards together with patients of other diagnoses. The resulting Boynton Report (Department of Health and Social Security 1980) painted a picture of a bleak, heavily routinized, strictly authoritarian hospital regime that heavily restricted patients' activities, organized the day to suit nursing shift patterns, and provided few opportunities for therapy of any sort. A total of 205 recommendations led to significant changes over the subsequent years. Following the deaths over a period of seven years of three black patients while they were held in seclusion at Broadmoor Hospital, another inquiry was initiated (Special Hospitals Service Authority 1993), the results of which were subsequently made public. This inquiry focused on the intensive care unit at Broadmoor, and uncovered a macho culture with a punitive use of medication, seclusion and other restrictions, lack of attention to the cultural needs of patients, all coupled with a sterile routinization of life on the ward and a depersonalization of patients in the eyes of staff. The outcome of this report was 47 recommendations and consequent changes to care at Broadmoor.

The most upsetting inquiry for anyone committed to the care of psychiatric patients was undoubtedly the Blom-Cooper Report. This inquiry was set up in response to yet another critical television documentary, alleging that patients' complaints were not properly dealt with at Ashworth Hospital. It revealed an uncaring and a demeaning attitude to patients, resulting in their harassment and bullying; a low quality of life for patients, provoking difficult to manage behaviour; substandard nursing care; substandard medical care; and substandard management. The main nursing union at that time was the Prison Officers Association (POA), which chose to instruct its members not to cooperate with the inquiry. Some of those who did give evidence were harassed, threatened and intimidated. Racist literature and posters were found on display in various parts of the hospital. A total of 90 recommendations were made.

The Blom-Cooper inquiry was something of a turning point for Ashworth and probably for the other High Security Psychiatric Hospitals also. An intensive, serious effort was made to implement the recommendations of the report at Ashworth. This resulted in the introduction of '24-hour care', a transformation that came to symbolize a change in culture and of attitude to patients. Prior to this, patients had been locked in their rooms at night; but with '24-hour care' patients were then free to leave their rooms at any time. A rigorous procedure was introduced that resulted in all patient complaints being taken seriously and carefully investigated. Following the inquiry the dominance of the POA over nurses in the High Security Hospitals was broken, and significant numbers left the POA to join alternative professional bodies and unions. Finally, it was in the wake of the Blom-Cooper Inquiry that the Ashworth PD unit was set up and opened as a ground-breaking, new way to provide therapeutic care to this difficult patient group.

It would be pleasant to be able to say at this point that the High Security services have gone from strength to strength, without further major difficulties. Unfortunately this is not the case: instead the focus of criticism has moved from the poor care described in the three reports, to poor security practices, and to controversy about the care of PD patients in particular. In 1996 a patient absconded from the Ashworth PD unit while on accompanied leave, and subsequently made allegations of paedophile activity on one of the wards, financial irregularities of various sorts, and the availability of pornography, drugs and alcohol. The paedophile activity was alleged to have taken place during the visits of a child and her father (himself an ex-patient) to one of the Ashworth wards. The subsequent public inquiry (the Fallon Report – Fallon *et al.* 1999) revealed that there were indeed a variety of financial 'scams' in operation on one ward, and that some videotaped pornography was available. Security rules were inconsistent and poorly implemented on the PD unit, searches of patients and their property were not routinely and uniformly undertaken, and visits to the ward were not properly monitored. The inquiry was not able finally to determine whether the child visitor had been abused, but concluded that it was a possibility. In the wake of the Fallon Report security was considerably tightened at all the High Security Hospitals: for example, random searching of patients was introduced; more detailed regulations about patients' personal property were put in place; computers were removed from patients' rooms; and all videotapes were reviewed to remove any possibility of the existence of pornography. A further review of security by Sir Richard Tilt, former Director General of the Prison Service (the Tilt Report – Tilt *et al.* 2000) led to the introduction of further security precautions, including a recommendation to end 24-hour care on admission wards.

At very much the same time (during 1998) Michael Stone was convicted of murdering a woman and her child who were out walking in the countryside. During the course of his trial it came to light that he suffered from a personality disorder, and had been rejected by psychiatric services on the grounds that his condition was untreatable. Considerable public criticism of psychiatry ensued. At the end of the millennium, therefore, the care of offenders with a personality disorder was a matter of public and political concern. Following a consultation exercise, the UK government proposed to set up a new service for people who are dangerous and severely personality disordered (DSPD), not prison or hospital, but midway between the two. Controversially the intention has been declared to bring in new Mental Health Act legislation to enable the preventive detention, before any crime has been committed, of those with DSPD.

All these events had an impact on the nurses who were the subjects of the research described in this book. They have, jointly, generally raised nurses' anxiety and caused feelings of insecurity. Psychiatric nurses who work with and care for personality disordered offenders are unsure about the future of their careers. They have continually to attend not only to what actually happens, but also to any negative interpretations that may be made in the eyes of others. They feel under public scrutiny much of time, with things as trivial as a patient's supervised leave sometimes attracting critical newspaper articles. They have also had to contend with continual changes of management and policy, changes in their own professional organizations politics, and the general changes in the National Health Service in the UK over the past 30 years. It is perhaps hardly surprising that some feel battered and demoralized.

Nursing care of PD

Little exists in the way of systematic descriptive research about the care of PD patients in the High Security Hospitals. Richman (1998) reports an ethnographic, participant observation study, conducted on one PD ward at Ashworth Hospital during 1988. This provides the sole empirically derived piece of work conducted by an objective observer into the daily life and functioning of this type of ward, usefully describing the patients' as well as the staff's points of view. Richman tells us how the patients believed both themselves and their ward to be 'special', a place where they had privileges in accord with this enhanced status. Thus patients believed that they had been able to block some admissions and transfers into the ward, and kept themselves together as an exclusive group within the hospital as a whole. They were willing and able to challenge the authority of the staff at every turn, whether this was in an attempt to stretch the ward regulations or assert their moral superiority over the staff. Staff were regarded by patients as being there for their benefit, and were made to work hard. For example, any attempt by staff to stretch their meal breaks would be met with urgent requests or a manufactured incident that demanded the nurses' presence. Nurses' loyalty and trustworthiness were tested by patients, who fed them confidences to see whether or not they were maintained. A clear patient hierarchy was visible, with two pairs of patients competing for leadership, with symbolic displays of power and status being regular events. According to Richman, nurses were valued by the PD patients not for their professional expertise, but because of their personal characteristics (e.g. openness, humour, non-judgemental attitude, physical prowess, honesty, etc.). Through Richman's eyes we gain insight into the realities of daily life for nurses and patients on a PD unit. Thus his account is rare and extremely valuable.

Since the work of Peplau, who brought the neo-Freudianism of Harry Stack Sullivan into the nursing literature in the 1950s, psychiatric nursing textbooks have given a dominant emphasis to the importance of the nurse–patient relationship. This emphasis has been well received by psychiatric nurses in the UK, as it harmonizes with the reality of their daily work with the mentally ill. It has been so frequently remarked as to become a truism, that nurses spend the most time with patients and therefore develop strong relationships with them. Nurse–patient relationships are seen in a variety of ways within the psychiatric nursing literature. In their formal derivation from neo-Freudianism by Peplau, such relationships are seen as a psychotherapeutic method in themselves. Others have interpreted them as being a necessary means of delivering nursing care, or a method of humane control of patients, particularly in relation to the prevention of violent incidents. At the very least, good nurse–patient relationships are necessary for a ward to operate harmoniously, making daily life together bearable and reasonably smooth.

Noak (1995) reflects some of these perspectives, and argues that a good nurse–patient relationship enables the nurse to become an advocate of the patient, and allows the nurse to get to know the patient well, thus developing empathy. He also argues that a good relationship assists the patient to become engaged with and committed to therapy, and provides interpersonal continuity and stability. He therefore appears to see the nurse–patient relationship as having a restorative or re-parenting function, as well as a means by which patients ambivalent about treatment may be engaged with the process using the leverage that a relationship supplies. These are laudable goals, but Noak cannot point to any empirical evidence that they can be accomplished, nor does he define in any detail exactly what constitutes an effective nurse–patient relationship with a person suffering from a personality disorder.

Noak (1995) identifies that the main threat to good nurse–patient relationships comes from the manipulative, rule-breaking, boundary pushing behaviour of PD patients. He suggests that this needs to be counteracted by nursing team consistency, multidisciplinary team support, and the recognition by managers of manipulative behaviour. Neilson (1991) also sees manipulative behaviour as a threat to therapeutic nurse–patient relationships, identifying the remedy as nursing team consistency. However he perceives PD patients as capable of a second means of upsetting and destabilising good nurse–patient relationships: splitting. He conceives of this in its psychodynamic sense as the projection of good and bad aspects of the self onto the nursing team. He goes on to describe how this can have two negative outcomes: (i) the production of sentimentalized and over-dependent good relationships with some staff; and (ii) the production of enmity, hostility and avoidance in and by other staff. Finally he argues that this can result in conflict within the team. His solution is that nurses need to encourage an open and accepting atmosphere for the team, and make good use of conflict resolution strategies.

The daily reality of nursing relationships with PD patients has nowhere been described better than by Melia et al. (1999). Due to the characteristics of the patients, relationships are highly charged and emotionally intense, with high levels of anger and hostility on their part towards nurses. The patients' expectation of harm and exploitation leads them to seize upon signs of behaviour on the part of the nurses indicating this, and results in recriminations, accusations, and loyalty testing behaviour. Thus they alternate between possessive and dismissive attitudes to the nurses. They blame others for their past actions and current predicament, seeking to recruit any sympathetic nurse to their point of view. Melia et al. do not cast 'splitting' in the same psychodynamic light as Neilson. Instead they view it as a number of related behaviours for which they offer no motivational explanation. The first of these is complaining to one member of staff about the actions of another, and the second is persuading individual staff to 'bend' the rules. The third is when a patient tries to create a special and secretive relationship with an individual member of staff. All produce team conflict that can be further exploited by patients. Melia *et al.* therefore see the nurse–patient relationship as a therapeutic tool whereby patients can learn, primarily via guided reality testing and feedback, a different psychosocial world view closer to that of everyday society.

For Melia *et al.* the solution to the problems and tensions generated within nurses' relationships with PD patients lies in the organization and structuring of nursing care. Ward-based nursing care has traditionally been task orientated, i.e. the ward has a set routine and a usual number of tasks to be undertaken during a nursing shift. These tasks are allocated to members of the nursing team by the nurse in charge who ensures that they are satisfactorily carried out. This method of ward organization declined in the 1970s and was replaced by primary nursing (Bowers 1989). This allocates the care of individual patients to individual nurses, and such care spans the shift system, thus encouraging the development of individualized nurse–patient relationships. Melia *et al.* consider that this approach isolates individual nurse–patient dyads and may accentuate the difficulties engendered by those with personality disorder. Thus they recommend the introduction of triumvirate nursing: a system whereby nurses work in teams of three, each with equal responsibility for nursing their patients. The three nurses then clinically supervise each other, providing support and objectivity via meetings of the triumvirate. Melia *et al.* do not therefore describe the therapeutic mechanics of using the nurse–patient relationship to achieve change and growth for PD patients. This is unfortunate as such descriptive nursing care information does not completely exist in the literature, and the authors so obviously do have this expertise. Instead they concentrate on how triumvirate nursing can be used to contain the patient and avoid the potentially negative outcomes of their methods of relating to the nurses. Valuable though this is, it is a defensive strategy that implies success to be the resistance of manipulation and splitting.

In an earlier paper by some of the same authors (Moran and Mason 1996), an attempt is made to describe what nurses should be 'doing' with PD patients. This description is a response to the fact that, while debate on the definition of PD and appropriate legal frameworks for care rumbles on, little actual guidance for nurses about 'doing nursing' exists. They therefore describe, based upon their own clinical experience, seven principles for nursing care. Some of these can usefully be viewed as ways in which the nurse–patient relationship can be therapeutically exploited for mutual benefit, others may be better perceived as attitudinal and belief prerequisites to the establishment of good relationships:

Usufruct – enjoy their dynamic   Instead of being threatened by the manipulation of PD patients, nurses should seek to enjoy and appreciate seeing through it. Moran and Mason go even further and hint that this enjoyment should be shared with the manipulating patient, thus allowing nurses and patients to work together constructively, rather than antagonistically, in defining the ward's rules.

Never be surprised   Sudden changes in the attitude and demeanour of PD patients should be met in the first instance without surprise or judgement. In fact Moran and Mason recommend no overt emotional reaction whatsoever. They view nurses' immediate emotional reactions (e.g. anger, disgust) as allowing an opening for patients to rush them into unwise decisions and statements. Instead they recommend that nurses should give themselves time to think carefully and calmly in order to arrive at a considered response.

Humour   Moran and Mason argue that humour can be used by nurses in a variety of ways: to tell uncomfortable truths without confrontation, to defuse tense situations and, when used in a self-deprecating way, to hinder patients' attempts to dominate nurses through ridicule.

99 per cent honesty   Moran and Mason recommend that nurses are honest to the point of discomfort with PD patients. Unfortunately they do not specify what nurses should be honest about, nor in what situations, while they do assert that patients will not, in the short term, like it.

Destabilizing the static   PD patients on a ward form into a fairly rigid hierarchy or dominance order. Moran and Mason suggest that it is the nurses' place to move up and down through different levels of this hierarchy, presumably by supporting patients at different times at different levels of the informal hierarchy, in order to break up entrenched patterns of dominance.

Rule flexibility   What Moran and Mason have to say here is ambiguous and difficult to understand. At one level they appear to be saying that nurses should assist patients in the legitimate breaching of rules, with the aim of destabilizing the patients' informal hierarchy. The difficulty is in defining what sort of rule bending is 'legitimate'. The necessity for the strict upholding of security rules, plus the Fallon Inquiry report on the disaster that ensues when they are not, makes this recommendation seem rather suspect.

Vulnerability   Nurses should wait for the moment when the PD patient needs them and approaches them with a specific request; then in fulfilling this request they can elicit gratitude and indebtedness from the patient. Moran and Mason suggest that this can then be used to build the relationship and enable the nurse to display altruism.

Interestingly, the nursing literature on PD care, such as it is, fails to mention or discuss core nursing rehabilitative functions. These have been a central part of the nursing role since the publications of, for example, Barton (1959). Either these approaches are not seen as relevant to the nursing care of PD, or it is not recognized that they require a specific application to patients of this sort. Neither is the use of the nursing process or nursing models discussed. Specific applications of these nursing technologies to the care of PD patients are absent from the literature. Nurses caring for PD patients on the ground are therefore left to grapple with the intricacies of making these things operate in a positively functional way within the context of their particular environment, whether that be an acute admission psychiatric ward, medium secure unit, mental illness ward of a High Security Hospital, or specialist PD unit in a high security setting.

The problem with all of the published literature is that it represents the voice of experience, clinical lore, tradition and wisdom, but not empirical evidence. Little exists, even in the way of systematic and objective descriptive research, to underpin the arguments, assertions and recommendations made in the published body of clinical nursing literature.

Noak (1995) lists forensic psychiatric nurses as being involved in the delivery of a number of therapies to PD patients. These include long-term individual psychotherapy, group psychotherapy, cognitive therapy, psychosexual counselling, and behaviour therapy. The literature on these therapies is diverse, but none of the nursing literature takes up the issue of how these are to be applied by nurses within their everyday practice of caring for patients. Thus the published literature makes it appear that nurses jump in and out of the role of 'psychotherapist' as group or individual sessions begin and end. How this is managed, how it overflows into daily nursing care, or into the general behaviour of patients, is not considered anywhere as a topic for discussion. Tennant and Hughes (1997) provide a case study that exemplifies a representative mix of therapeutic interventions. Eight sessions are named in the care plan, seven of which are individual or group therapeutic sessions. Only one has any reference to daily life on the ward, and even that makes no mention of how the patient is to be managed within the context of the ward community. In a second paper, Tennant and Hughes (1998) describe the use of a 'men's group' with violent PD offenders, focusing on dysfunctional concepts of masculinity, and Aiken and Sharp (1997) describe a psychodynamic psychotherapy group which, again, is described separately from daily nursing care. Only the TC literature (e.g. Yurkovich 1989) makes clear how, by that model, 'therapy' and 'nursing' can be an integrated whole. A rare exception to this is a study by Cremin et al. (1995) that describes how a psychodynamically informed style of interaction can be incorporated into everyday nursing with impulsive, self-harming, PD patients. The study was of an extremely small sample (four cases), but did produce results suggesting that nursing interactions can reduce self-harming behaviour.

A number of factors may influence the degree to which psychiatric nurses become involved in formal psychotherapeutic approaches. The constraints of staffing shortages and the shift rotation system may make it difficult for nurses to be involved at all. Secondly, these therapeutic skills are difficult for nurses to acquire, and are not taught in any depth during basic nurse training. Hence only the most keen and dedicated nurses manage to secure sufficient training to play a lead role in formal therapy. Lastly, inter-disciplinary conflict and competition between the psychiatric professions may make it hard for nurses to gain access to groups as co-therapists, or for them to gain high-quality supervision and/or recognition for their work. None of these practical factors is comprehensively discussed in the nursing literature about PD care, although some are mentioned in descriptive and exploratory research about psychiatric nursing in general. The only paper that addresses the training issues is that by Hughes and Tennant (1996), who describe how three differing levels of training in cognitive-behavioural interventions were delivered to PD unit nursing staff at Rampton Hospital. These authors sensibly tackle the practical issues involved in this type of exercise.

In the UK High Security Hospitals psychiatric nurses are responsible for security as well as the therapeutic aspects of care. This has been discussed at length by Burrow (1991, 1998), who describes how nurses keep doors locked, search wards, rooms and patients, monitor mail, telephone calls and visitors, escort patients to different parts of the hospital, and manage parole systems. The requirement to rigorously operate such systems when they are disliked and rejected by patients is a hindrance to the formulation of adult-to-adult relationships between nurses and patients, and makes it difficult for nurses to act in any way as patient advocates. However it may be that this debate has been overblown in relation to forensic psychiatric nurses, as all psychiatric nurses working in acute care have responsibilities for security, albeit of a lesser intensity, in general hospital settings. In any case, Burrow (1998) recommends that therapy and security can be melded in nursing practice if security is stated in terms of patient care.

Thus the nurses' role with PD patients in the High Security Hospitals can therefore be seen as threefold. They manage the daily care, organization, activity and routine of patients. Sometimes as part of that daily routine, and sometimes separately from it, they provide individual or group-oriented therapeutic interventions to patients. Lastly, they are responsible for security – keeping patients in the hospital, and preventing them from harming others or themselves while they reside there. These three tasks can sometimes sit uneasily together.

This research study

The study reported on in this book aimed to identify the factors underlying and maintaining nurses' positive therapeutic attitudes to patients with severe

PD, in order to inform a support and training strategy to nurture such attitudes. The author had noticed that, despite prevailing negative attitudes towards people with PD, some psychiatric professionals managed to keep to a positive approach over a long period of time. How those professionals did that, therefore, surfaced as an important question. If it was possible to discover the cognitive strategies used by those professionals in the face of the difficult behaviours of PD patients, it might be possible to share those with others or train them in their use. Further questions of interest were how attitudes related to the age, experience, gender and grade of nurse, whether individual hospitals had individual and discrete cultures in relation to the care of PD patients, and how attitudes were related to the ethical stance of the professionals.

In order to answer these questions, all nurses working in the three English High Security Hospitals ($n = 2,503$) were sent a questionnaire on their attitude to PD patients and beliefs about them. In addition, a random sample of 121 nurses, stratified for hospital, grade and work area, were interviewed on the topic.

No previously developed scale on attitude to PD was available. The rating of nursing attitude used in the Miller and Davenport (1996) study remains unpublished and it has not been possible to obtain a copy. Lewis and Appleby (1988) developed their own 22-item semantic differential scale to be used in conjunction with a variety of forms of the same case history, but this was not suitable for distribution in a large-scale survey. The only other research scale that has endeavoured to assess staff's emotional response to difficult patients is the Hospital Treatment Rating Scale (HTRS, Colson et al. 1986). Published psychometric data on this scale is incomplete, and it consists of several subsections with different properties. However, its use in long-term psychiatric care settings has revealed that staff consider patients with 'character pathology' to be particularly difficult.

A new questionnaire, adapted and derived from the HTRS, was therefore created: the Attitude to Personality Disorder Questionnaire (APDQ). This was piloted with a convenience sample of local psychiatric nurses, following which the number of items was reduced and some rephrased. These were then sent out to all nursing staff in the three hospitals.

Staff lists were provided by each hospital's personnel department. Questionnaires were distributed, in individually addressed envelopes containing reply-paid envelopes, to every nurse in each High Security Hospital six weeks prior to the interviews. Returned questionnaires were not individually identifiable, so personalized follow-up to non-responders could not be conducted. It was decided that ensuring the anonymity of respondents was more critical to the response rate than the potential to send reminders. As an alternative, bundles of duplicate questionnaires were delivered to each of the wards by the research assistants at the same time as they were conducting the interviews.

The overall response rate was 26 per cent – a relatively low response rate that is typical for research in the High Security Hospitals. In order to assess for non-response bias, the gender and grade mix of the responders was compared to that of the non-responders. This analysis indicated that the responders were representative with respect to gender but that there was a particularly low rate of response for unqualified staff. PD unit nurses had a much better response rate, but this cannot be precisely calculated because the survey nurses were asked to define for themselves whether they worked on a PD unit or not. These self-definitions probably do not precisely match those used by the research team. The better response of PD unit nurses means that the survey is well representative of their views. The refusal rate for the interviews was less than 10 per cent, and the range of attitude to PD measured from those interviews matches accurately the variation in questionnaire responses by hospital, grade and gender. This implies that, even though the questionnaire response rate was low, the sample obtained was representative.

Semi-structured interview schedules were developed, based upon a litera-ture review and the theoretical thinking of the research team. Additional items and changes were offered by the project steering group. Both research assistants used this preliminary schedule with four volunteers from within the Department of Mental Health Nursing at City University, following which additional changes to the schedule were made. Once finalized, the interview schedule was not altered in order to maintain consistency of responses and comparability between hospitals.

Both research assistants recruited to the project had previous training and experience of conducting research interviews. Additional individual training was given. The interview schedule was piloted with five members of the University with experience of working with PD clients, in order to perfect the schedule and develop the interviewing skills of the researchers. The senior researcher, who had considerable experience in fieldworker training, gave individual feedback on style and follow-up questions to the research assistants. In order to improve parity of interviewing styles the researchers interviewed each other, and listened to each other's interviews on tape.

Consistency between the two interviewers was attained by training them together:

- pilot interviews were conducted in the presence of the other research assistant;
- during the data collection period at each hospital, the research assistants discussed in detail the way their interviews were progressing, how replies to each question were working out, and listened to tapes of each other's interviews;
- following each site visit, interview transcripts were examined by the project leader, who gave feedback to the research assistants together.

Following the obtaining of staff lists from the hospitals it was discovered that standard stratified random sampling for PD unit and non-PD unit staff would yield only very low numbers of staff from the PD units, because the numbers of staff working in those units formed only a small percentage of the total. As the purpose of the research was to identify the factors that support positive long-term attitudes to PD, it was decided to take roughly half the sample from the pool of PD unit staff. Stratification proportional to grade was maintained. Both night and day nursing staff were interviewed, with interviews being conducted at night when necessary.

All 121 interviews were tape recorded and fully transcribed. Following transcription, each tape was listened to by members of the research team and any inaccuracies or errors in the transcript were corrected. In order to facilitate coding and analysis of the data, all transcripts were imported into qualitative data analysis software (QSR.NUD.IST version 4). All 121 inter-views were coded by one researcher on overall attitude to PD, using the dimensions of analysis provided by the factor analysis of the APDQ. A random sample of 30 of these were independently coded by another researcher (blind to the initial ratings) using the same method, yielding an intraclass correlation coefficient of 0.96.

Responses to individual questions were collected and analysed together. As some topics spanned several questions, or material on some topics was spread throughout the interviews, analysis via question responses was sup-plemented (and in some cases replaced) by text word searches. The material thus gathered was read, and then coded into appropriate categories before being finally analysed and described. Categories of content or of responses to individual questions were quantified and related to overall attitude to PD, using contingency table analysis.

The attitudes of nurses

The response rate to the survey was 26 per cent (651 nurses), and the largest single group of respondents were in their thirties, with relatively few in their twenties. This would appear to indicate a fairly mature mix of staff, given that entry to nurse training is conventionally in the late teens and early twenties. There were roughly two male nurses to every female nurse working in the High Security Hospitals. Most nurses (61 per cent) had worked outside the High Security Hospital system at some stage in their previous careers. These hospitals cannot therefore be seen as static closed institutions and must be open to change and influence from outside. Most staff had a rela-tively small amount of experience of working in the High Security Hospitals (under five years). Turnover is highest among unqualified staff, with 82 per cent having less than five years' experience, compared to 39 per cent of basic grade trained nurses.

Most nurses viewed PD patients as a difficult patient group to care for and treat. Less than 1 in 10 nurses considered them to pose no or mild difficulties. The large majority of nurses considered that PD patients would not engage with treatment or have a good outcome. Less than 1 in 5 nurses expressed any optimism about the treatment of PD patients.

Although the balance of opinion was that PD patients should continue to be cared for in High Security Hospital settings, there was considerable divergence and little sign of any consensus among nurses on this issue. There was strong support from nurses that PD patients should be cared for in specialist wards (more than 70 per cent of respondents). That this opinion was expressed against the backdrop of the ongoing Fallon Inquiry makes this finding even more striking. It may be that large numbers of nurses simply want PD patients cared for elsewhere – if not in prison then in a separate part of the hospital.

Most nurses felt unprepared and less well trained to work with PD patients. However the situation was not completely bleak, as 1 in 4 nurses did consider that they had been adequately trained. Those working on the PD units were more likely to indicate that they considered themselves adequately trained (30 per cent), in comparison to those who worked on other types of ward.

On nearly all questionnaire items, Rampton staff were the most positive and Ashworth staff the least. Although the reason for this is not known, there are several possibilities. The ongoing Fallon Inquiry at the time of the study may have led to more pessimistic attitudes at Ashworth. Other possible explanations were: (1) Rampton PD unit staff volunteered to work with the PD client group, whereas Ashworth nurses were allocated to work there at the time it was opened; (2) the Rampton unit was only recently opened and at an enthusiastic stage; and (3) the different hospitals had accumulated differing groups of PD patients.

Female nursing staff were more optimistic about the treatment of PD, and were less likely to think prison more appropriate. They also considered themselves better trained for the care and treatment of PD patients than the male nurses. In a similar way, the higher grades of nurses were more positive towards PD patients. Experience of working on a dedicated unit for PD also clearly had an impact on attitude, as PD unit nurses had a more positive attitude than those working in other parts of the hospitals.

Interestingly, those who had worked as nurses (qualified or unqualified) outside the High Security Hospital system were more likely to regard the care and treatment of PD patients as difficult, were less likely to rate team-work with PD patients as good, and are less likely to consider themselves well trained to work with PD patients. This would appear to indicate that attitudes towards PD outside of the forensic psychiatric system are even worse than those within.

Principal components analysis of the responses to the affective statements in the questionnaire revealed five components:

- Enjoyment/loathing
- Security/vulnerability
- Acceptance/rejection
- Purpose/futility
- Enthusiasm/exhaustion

PD unit nurses report greater enjoyment and purpose, older nurses greater exhaustion.

Summary

This chapter has described the differing organization of care for PD patients in each of the three English High Security Psychiatric Hospitals, and how that has led to differing patient populations as well as different approaches to treatment. The way in which PD care in the UK has developed over time has also been shown to be intrinsically tied up with a series of scandals and public inquiries into forensic psychiatric care. Those same inquiries set the context for nurses' experience of caring for PD patients in these settings, accentuating feelings of vulnerability, and susceptibility to public scrutiny and criticism. All this is overlaid upon the general negative attitudes towards PD patients of all the psychiatric professions described in the first chapter. Within this situation the nursing role is to provide and manage the daily routine of patient care and life in hospital, provide psychotherapy of one sort or another (although the involvement of nurses in therapy is ambiguous and variable), and maintain the security of care. It is hardly surprising, therefore, that the initial survey reported here confirmed that, in general, attitudes to PD patients were negative, and nurses felt poorly prepared to manage their behaviour.

However, the survey also illuminated the components of positive and negative attitudes to PD patients. Having a positive attitude means that the nurses concerned enjoy their work, feel secure, willingly accept PD patients, have a sense of purpose and enthusiasm. Vice versa, the negative attitude nurses tend to loath their work, feel vulnerable, do not willingly accept PD patients, feel that they are wasting their time and feel exhausted. Subsequent chapters will demonstrate exactly how these positive or negative attitudes arise and are maintained over time, and what impact they have upon nurses and the care they provide to patients.

3   Trials and tribulations

Caring for PD patients is not an easy task. They are generally considered to be difficult patients by all psychiatric professionals at every level of service. Even those treated as outpatients are considered hard to care for, let alone those whose condition is so severe and associated with such criminal behaviour that they are residing within the High Security Hospitals. In this chapter the problems faced by staff in managing and caring for PD patients will be described. The crimes committed by patients evoke emotional reactions from staff. In addition the nurses who were interviewed described five aspects of the behaviour of PD patients that contribute to making them 'difficult': manipulation, self-harm, violence, complaints, and their tendency to form among themselves an informal and exploitative hierarchy within the ward.

These behaviours have a profound impact upon nurses. The level of manipulative behaviour deployed by the patients is pervasive, complex, subtle, and skilled, to the degree that nurses can sometimes admire its artistry, even when suffering from the consequences. The extent and nature of self-harm can elicit feelings of nausea and repugnance. The violent behaviour of patients, although not necessarily frequent, can be severe, and has led to nurses taking retirement on medical grounds. The use to which PD patients put the official complaints procedure can put nurses under enormous and crippling stress, especially within the context of a service that has been put under the microscope by a string of highly public inquiries, and frequently features in national newspapers. These are just a few of the things that make PD patients difficult, and explain why they are such an unpopular group of patients that evoke feelings of pessimism, despair, anger and dislike throughout the psychiatric system.

Bad, evil and monstrous

In considering this topic, it is important to realize how serious and reprehensible are the crimes of those committed to the High Security Hospitals. Although not every patient has committed very serious crimes, many have.

The index offences (the crimes resulting in their committal to the High Security Hospitals) of these patients involve rape with severe violence, murder, torture and mutilation of children (including taking photographs of the event), necrophilia, post-mortem dismemberment, cannibalism, etc. Interviewees described a number of such events, and even at the distance of reading transcripts of interviews, these are significantly emotionally shocking.

There were some staff who endorsed the use of the words bad, evil and monstrous in describing PD patients: *Evil, yes. Bad, definitely. Monstrous, maybe one or two.* Even those who rejected the terminology sometimes admitted to having feelings like this: *They're not appropriate but I'd be a hypocrite if I didn't say that I didn't think them sometimes! There's some days and there's some times when you're reading somebody's background and criminal history that you, that those words might enter your head. You perhaps wouldn't say them out loud, but . . .* However, others rejected the terminology outright as completely inappropriate.

One of the factors that determined whether staff considered a patient evil or not was the nature of their crime, and how it was interpreted or perceived. The more severe or serious the index offence, the more likely the patient is to be called evil or monstrous. For some nurses this meant patients who had murdered, as opposed to those who had not. Other nurses were more non-specific, referring only to barbaric or horrible crimes as a reason for using these words. Of those nurses who were specific, it was clear that the degree of vulnerability of the victims was important, thus crimes against women or children attracted particular disapprobation: *You're talking about paedophiles, rapists, people who harm their babies, yeah I think they are quite adequate terms.* Use of torture or any form of sadism evoked similar reactions from nurses: *I see people get sexually excited at the thought of attempted murder and being part of it really, their faces, I couldn't describe looks, evil, evil.* Any indication that the patients were in control of themselves at the time of the offence was also taken as an indicator that they could be considered evil; for example, if the violence was planned in advance rather than being impulsive. In this context a nurse described how a patient had carefully planned to kill a member of staff, preparing a knife in the workshop, built in three parts, each brought back to the ward and concealed, and then waited for the targeted member of staff to be in a vulnerable situation. This entire process had taken at least two months of careful planning, preparation and execution. In this case the plan was discovered and a potentially fatal incident averted. However, that planning element is taken by some nurses to be indicative of 'evil'. *They go that extra yard, the torture element and the consistent element, the hunting down of people and the preying on certain victims over long periods of time. This is not a sort of anger.*

For others any sense that patients were responsible for their actions, or 'knew what they were doing' was enough for them to be thought of as evil.

For some nurses, patients with an abuse history could at least in some way be understood if not exonerated. But those patients who did not have a history of being abused during childhood were more likely to be perceived as having no excuse and therefore to be evil: *If they say he has a good upbringing, didn't come from a broken home, he wasn't battered, he wasn't raped, he wasn't done anything, he had a good life . . . and committed a hideous crime, then . . .* Patients who refused to accept that what they had done was wrong, showed no remorse, or refused any treatment were also likely to attract the label of evil or monster: *But he was an evil man. He took no responsibility for his actions. And he felt he could do what he wanted, and he didn't care what he had done. No apparent remorse for what he had done to these children.* Some nurses pointed to the contrast between the apparent normality of the patient – who appears to be an ordinary nice kind of person, laughing and joking with others on the ward – and the crime committed. The sense of dissonance, of something not being quite right, or the sense of something being kept hidden underneath or controlled, makes some nurses consider the patient as evil: *You know it can, I mean she can be evil to others, evil to herself, the staff. And another night I could come in and she's so pleasant and nice.*

In short, PD patients were most likely to attract these negative labels if:

- they had not been abused as children
- their index offence had been serious violence against vulnerable victims
- their offence had been planned in advance, and involved torture
- they refused treatment in hospital
- they showed no remorse
- they appeared to be nice people.

Nurses had several theories about why the terminology of evil had currency. The largest proportion (20 per cent of the total) blamed the media, particularly newspapers, for portraying patients in this way. This was acknowledged to be a double influence. It was formative of the expectations of people before they entered nursing, and it continued to shape them thereafter: *Because nurses are human anyhow, you know we are receptive to outside influences and people who have never actually had to work with PDs get the image of, how can I put this without . . . that all PDs are monsters. Because of what is written about them in the Press.* The actions of the Press were seen by nurses as being sensationalist, directed solely at selling more newspapers, and on the whole unhelpful. Nurses made similar criticisms (although less frequently) about the statements of judges at trials: *A lot of these are bandied about – these words – by the defence and the prosecution, before it even gets to the judge. The judge can mention something to a jury as I say in his summary . . . but I don't believe that once they are in the system, that you should use words like that.*

Nurses characterized the terminology of evil as an emotional rather than considered and objective response to their PD patients. One nurse likened the use of these words to swearing, in that they are a way for the inarticulate to express their feelings. The emotion is not named by all the respondents, but those that do, label it as anger. Evidence that anger is the emotion in view is underlined by the associated use of other emotion-laden terms, e.g. 'murdering bastard', 'inflammatory expressions', 'parasite to society', 'leeches', 'atrocity', 'very emotive', 'very provocative', etc.

A few nurses suggested that people were willing to use the terminology of evil because it made the patients who do such terrible things appear wholly different and non-human: *It's easier to label people as – and maybe it's safer to think that they are a different species, that they are not human beings like us, like me and you. Maybe it's sort of more comfortable to think that. That they are monsters and they are not like us, but I think maybe people are frightened that maybe we've all got that element in with us, we're all sort of human beings at the end of the day.*

Religious explanations of narratives around evil were almost completely absent from the interviews. Only one nurse made reference to 'Satanism', and then only in the context of saying that index offences involving satanic practices were, for him, an indicator that the patient was evil. No nurses talk about evil being a compelling external force, or talk in Christian, Manicheean, or other metaphysical ways about the nature of evil or demonically offered temptation. The only other mentions of religion by nurses in this context were in relation to the moral choices they had made to work in forensic psychiatric services. It would appear that nurses are either a completely atheistic/humanistic group of people, or at the very least have no time, or can find no worthwhile place in their work, for such philosophies. There are nurses with a negative overall attitude to PD patients, who feel no liking for them, fear them, consider them a waste of time and call them 'evil monsters'. However these nurses do not engage in metaphysical theorizing about PD patients or their deeds. Instead, the word *evil* as used by these nurses seems to refer more simply to acts that are bad in the extreme.

The findings in this study partially replicate those of Mercer *et al.* (1999) and Richman (1999). These authors asked a sample of High Security Hospital nurses to comment on vignettes describing patients and their crimes. In common with this study, they found that patients were likely to be considered evil when crimes had been planned in advance and the victims were from vulnerable groups. In addition, because they included a wide range of examples in their vignettes, they discovered that PD patients were more likely to be considered evil than psychotic patients.

Reading about crimes of horror

In all three hospitals the case notes available on the wards contained clinical records, index offence histories and case conference reports. Clinical records could contain detailed analyses of offences and offending behaviour. The full record of the index offence, including depositions and photographs, was held centrally at medical records. Nurses would need to take time away from the ward, and have the authorization of the ward manager or responsible medical officer to access these records, sometimes referred to in the interviews as the 'black notes'. Two to three years previous to the research, the contents of the 'black notes' were held at ward level in some cases, and were more accessible to nursing staff. Reading these notes, hence being forced to confront the details of patients' crimes, could sometimes arouse strong feelings.

The largest groups of staff said they had become hardened to the reality of what patients had done, or were completely unaffected by it. A number of nurses who made these comments said they had become more hardened and less affected over time, and some even questioned whether this was a good personal development for them. *But because I'm aware that you can become inured to it, I try to take steps to make sure that I do keep a hold on reality.* Those who reported being currently unaffected were able to describe well the impact of this experience; how they were at first shocked by what had now become a matter of routine. Others who asserted that they were unaffected went on to describe, when pressed a little harder, an emotional response – typically when asked whether they ever thought about the victims. Yet others remarked that the victims of these crimes were unreal to them and thus evoked no emotion, either because they were strangers rather than people they had known, or because they were only represented by paper records.

> *What's happened to complete strangers doesn't affect me all that much.*

> *They are just words on a piece of paper and it doesn't affect me.*

> *If I saw it happen – different, but it's, it's written in a file it just, no.*

> *But they are faceless shadows really, you've not known them, you've never seen them, you don't know what they look like.*

The most common emotional reaction among staff was to feel angry about the crimes patients had committed, with 30 per cent of staff admitting to having felt this way at some point. *I can run the whole gauntlet of emotions from disgust, anger, I think possibly at times I may even hate people.* For some nurses anger is easily elicited when reading the case notes; for others this occurs when the patient is relating an index offence. *They're sitting describing it all, you know, I did this to them and I did that to them and your stomach's turning as you're doing it but you've still got to carry on and do it and you go out and think, fuck, I want to go in and kill him.* This anger may be directly about the index offence, at other times it is the contrast between the relatively good life that patients lead and the fact of what they have done that makes nurses feel angry. *I think, you know, people outside have lost loved ones, you know, you've destroyed lives of people who have been abused and raped, and things like this. But I mean they're happy, they're, run the bingo, the dances, they just carry on, you know, they have four meals a day.* It is, of course, this same angry contrast that generates headlines in newspapers from time to time. Alternatively, the index offence can be recalled and contrasted with the demands and criticisms a patient makes, thus eliciting anger. The interviewees spoke of angry feelings rising to the surface on days when patients complained, criticized, and moaned continually. For yet others the contrast that arouses anger is that between the amount of care and resources being delivered to the perpetrators of the crime, while the victims receive little or no help. In the words of one nurse: *Well I just think everything stinks way things go round, you know.* The nurses pointed out that it was especially difficult for those with families and young children to accept crimes such as paedophilia and child murder, and that these crimes in particular could elicit strong angry reactions. One respondent very clearly described the impact that having his first child had on his attitudes. Prior to the birth he was able to work relatively easily with patients who had committed this type of crime. However, once his baby was born his feelings underwent an enormous transformation. He found it difficult to come into work, and when there he didn't want to talk to these patients because he was so overcome with anger towards them. This nurse did work through these feelings with the help and support of his colleagues, but his response indicates the depth of anger and outrage that staff, as normal everyday moral people, can feel towards PD patients. Although nearly all nurses who expressed anger reported that they managed to contain these feelings, conceal them and act in a professional manner towards patients, it does seem likely that the feelings would manifest themselves somehow, either verbally or non-verbally. One nurse described his experience: *I sometimes wonder if patients here have a go at you and they say, you are keeping me locked up here doing this, if sometimes yeah, and you confront them and say, well did you ever think about the girl you raped or bloke you slashed, do you ever think about the family that, you know, that you broke into and killed the mother or the father and left the kids?* Expression of anger in relation to the index offences of PD patients was associated with an overall negative attitude to PD. This seems to contradict psychodynamic theory, which suggests that those who express their emotions and are knowledgeable about them will be more able to manage them positively.

Another common response was that of sadness. Feelings of compassion were expressed towards the victim, the victim's family, and the patient's family who were commonly perceived as also being devastated by the event. *I suppose it makes you feel sad really. You know whichever person it may be, that could be a life that's been spoiled and tainted. You know that person's direction in life's changed, hasn't it?* Nurses, when asked their thoughts about the victims, readily expressed these feelings of hurt and sorrow.

Fear was expressed in a number of different ways. It may be fear of the patients once the details of their index offences are known. *Somewhere at the back of your mind you never forget, you can't, not in a hospital like this because, I mean, okay I ain't going to be, well I could be raped, but you're going to get the guys who will beat you up, they will carry a chib on the ward, you know a blade or anything like that. I've got this inordinate fear of being slashed and it worries me more than being raped on the ward.* Nurses with this sort of reaction tend to be more cautious at work, and more aware of the need to keep themselves safe. That fear can also spill over into the personal and family life of nurses when they are outside the hospital. In this case the fear can be personal and about their own safety. *It's probably there all the time . . . even when I've gone out and been up an alleyway to this public house I go to I've got my fist clench with my keys in between my fingers in case somebody jumps out at me.* Or it can be fear for the safety of their family, and in this respect most of the nurses talked about being very protective of their children, suspecting people of holding harmful intentions or perverse desires towards them. Some of the nurses spoke of this being on their mind at all times. Other nurses were deeply affected differently by reading the case notes, and were unable to shrug off their feelings easily. They found the details haunting, had intrusive thoughts about them, and a few reported having nightmares.

Incomprehension was also common. Staff found it hard to comprehend just how anyone, whatever their upbringing or circumstances, could do the things that the patients had done. Different aspects of the index offence generated incomprehension for different nurses. It might be the savagery involved (e.g. multiple stab wounds, mutilation of the body), or the vulnerability of the victims (e.g. children), or the fact that victims were close members of the perpetrator's own family (e.g. parents or siblings). Some nurses made a contrast between psychotic patients, whose crimes could be understood in terms of their symptoms, and PD patients, whose crimes were more difficult, if not impossible, to grasp. In these cases it was the lack of feeling – the coldness and calculation involved, the lack of remorse and the tendency of PD patients to blame the victims – that nurses simply could not accept or empathize with. *I was talking to a lad that was, he was, in for multiple rape and he was explaining to me how a* [age deleted] *year old girl had lured him and asked to be sort of molested and then accused him later on. And how a girl . . . was – again – asking to be sort of raped even though he went over and assaulted her . . . and quite savagely raped her. He was sort of, he was still, it was her fault . . . that's quite difficult to understand.* In other cases the difficulty was in putting together the social reality of the patient as an apparently warm, humane individual, and what he had done. *But I've certainly met the people before I've been able to get through the notes, and, and I haven't been able to put it together, the person, and then I read about what they've done and I thought god, you know I find that hard to believe really.*

Alongside incomprehension, some nurses also felt, on occasion, revolted by what patients had done. This was expressed in words like 'horrific', 'horrendous', 'repulsed', 'disgusted', or 'revulsion'. These feelings were elicited by factors similar to incomprehension: savagery of the attack; vulnerability of the victim; coldness of the perpetrator; and lack of remorse. These feelings can be very strong and acute. *I was sat down and given a set of case notes, of a man who had committed a specifically horrific assault on his own son, on his own daughter. In which that child actually died, but it was the manner in which the child died and what was going on in their home at the time, that was the part of the revulsion as much as the death. It was the manner in which it was executed, the manner in his total lack of concern and consideration, for that child.* Another staff member reported how a colleague had gone to read the case notes about a patient who had killed his family, and on returning to the ward had vomited in the toilet and had to go home sick. In the course of the interviews nurses sometimes spoke with horror about some of the things their patients had done. Even at one remove, as a researcher, tales of children being tortured for personal gratification proved shocking and distressing.

In addition to the differentiated feelings described above, nurses also talked about being upset. This seemed to be a general term for a combination of feelings that have been described more specifically already, particularly sadness, anger, fear and revulsion. Nurses also spoke of feeling guilty for ignoring what patients had done, for setting aside their natural negative feelings and delivering nursing care to patients. Other nurses felt that knowledge of the index offence was burdensome, and placed them under stress and pressure, without being able to articulate quite why this was so. *Because at the back of our minds we know, we know that for instance on this ward that some even have killed and have committed some terrible crimes on children. Some of the most unimaginable things. And that that's there. That's there and that in itself is very very stressful. And I don't think we talk about it enough in this system. The reason we don't talk about it enough is because, you know, if you take a lid off, you know, everything goes all over the place. And I think that many nurses have to keep a tight lip and in order to do that.* Two other nurses mentioned that their feelings changed from day to day, swinging between acceptance of patients and rejection, depending on the current behaviour and attitude of the patient.

Devious, deceitful and manipulative

On top of the feelings aroused by the crimes committed by PD patients prior to their arrival in the High Security Hospital, staff also have to deal with the many difficult behaviours of patients once they are there. The most frequently mentioned was manipulation. Manipulation was something that staff brought up in relation to a number of issues, although the interview did not specifically ask about it. One of the most frequent ideas was that PD patients are manipulative; this might be a trait, characteristic, part of their personality, a result of upbringing, etc., but that is what they are.

It was a word that regularly appeared when nurses were asked 'What have you learned about nursing people with PD?' *Well I've learnt, obviously signs, there's obviously signs, symptoms and traits, of a psychopath. You, you, you learn to look out for. I mean a lot of cases sort of, do unsociable behaviour and, manipulative behaviour.* Three-quarters of the staff interviewed had something to say about manipulation.

There is no generally agreed definition of manipulation. However the interviewees' description of the manipulative behaviour of patients showed that, as used by nurses in the High Security Hospitals, the word means 'action to achieve a desired goal' (perverse or normal, symbolic or real) using deception, coercion and trickery, without regard for the interests or needs of those used in the process. Further classification of the behaviour called 'manipulative' showed there to be six different subtypes. Any one manipulative course of action by a patient may combine these elements in different and sometimes unique ways. Patients may use these methods as individuals, but they may also work cooperatively together as a group to manipulate staff and achieve their ends. Information about people is power, thus a foundation of many manipulative strategies is information about nurses, their opinions, families, likes and dislikes, interests, foibles, past decisions and actions, etc. Again this information may be compiled individually, or may be the collaborative project of several patients. Patients deploy these behavioural strategies against a wide range of targets, and against each other in order to achieve some sort of advantage.

Bullying

This incorporated a variety of methods used to exert pressure on nurses to comply with patients' expressed wishes and desires. At the mildest end of the spectrum this consisted of the constant repetition of requests. Nurses also recognized, as part of this process, a ratcheting mechanism. Once one small concession had been made, it would be immediately exploited and followed by more constant repetitious demands. *One moment they were asking for some tea, then they were asking for sandwich, and at 3 o'clock in the morning they were asking for bread to make toast.* The nurses' descriptions convey a sense of continuous pressure: they felt pushed, worn down, ground down and badgered by patients who persistently insisted on more all the time, and were not even willing to wait for their demands to be met. In the knowledge that saying 'No' could sometimes precipitate actual violent attack by the patient, nurses found the sheer constant pressure mentally draining and intimidating.

Further pressure came from the constant questioning and challenging attitude of patients. They engaged nurses in verbal debate and argument about the regulatory structure of the ward or hospital. They demanded parity with other patients on the ward or elsewhere in the system, or asked for the rules to be justified, and when the reason was given, they argued that it was invalid.

They cited examples of inconsistency between nurses, or by the same nurse at different times, as grounds for a rule to be relaxed. Alternatively, they argued from an external frame of reference – for example, ethical first principles, human rights, the Mental Health Act Code of Practice, the Patients' Charter, etc. In comparison to psychotic patients, PD patients were perceived to be articulate, and well able to express their views. They studied the rules, memorized them, and were able to twist them, in argument with the nurses, to suit their purposes to the degree that nurses could come to doubt themselves: *They have a habit of making you judge your own judgement about things. If you make a decision and say 'No you can't have that', they have got a habit then that they'll argue until the argument cannot go any further, and you sort of think about it... and say 'Oh I was being petty'.* Because patients studied the issues intensely, they found loopholes, grey areas, flaws in the rationale for rules, or issues not covered by existing rules, and exploited them to the full. All this was experienced by nurses as overpowering, a feeling of being embattled, having always to take the flak. *When they're told No, they can't have something, immediately that triggers a reaction from them, and they want to know why and they question and question, and for you to get in this argument with them you're wasting your time because you can be there all day, ... you get into a mind game with them and you can be there ten, fifteen minutes, and sometimes they're a lot cleverer than what we are with these mind games, ... you can't win at it.*

A process of incremental erosion was also described. Patients sought greater and greater liberties by first breaking or extending the limits of minor rules, then continuing the process, or waiting to see whether the nurses would respond and repeating the infraction. In this way the regulatory structure of the ward was gradually dissolved, and the nurses could lose control. One example given was of a patient who took over one of the ward interview rooms, slowly but surely converting it into a rest room, moving in a stereo, then a chair, and eventually his personal belongings. The first concession was said by nurses to be the thin end of the wedge – for example, running recreations a little over time, allowing patients to stay up a bit later, keeping the kitchen open a little longer. Patients then slowly extend and widen these concessions until it is clear that control has been completely lost, and the timetable of events is in their hands. Alternatively a similar process could be applied to rules. A patient may test the water by smoking in the wrong area to see how the staff would respond, or may exact what is ostensibly a one-off extension to the rule and make it a regular occurrence. Simple non-cooperation is another means by which patients can challenge the structure of the ward. All these efforts are felt by nurses to be a form of attack, as though patients are constantly testing them or trying to 'chisel away' at the rules the nurses are charged with upholding.

Outright rebellion or group pressure was an additional concern. All the above strategies could also be used by patients in a group, and were then seen as more threatening by staff. Examples were given of patients organizing 'sit-ins', breaking rules together and thus raising the stakes for any nurse to confront them, getting together to verbally challenge or question a nurse on the justification for a rule, and other orchestrated attempts to intimidate staff. Occasionally, individual staff members were singled out by patients for attack: they could pick on the nurse's perceived physical or behavioural deficits, have recourse to intense and repeated verbal abuse, or employ constant sarcasm to wear the nurse down. Alternatively, verbal means of exerting pressure were sometimes accompanied by non-verbal intimidation. For example, they were reported to: initiate conversations while standing over the sitting nurse; stare threateningly; follow nurses around; invade their personal space; develop a powerful, strong physique; prowl round the ward at night. By themselves these poses seem trivial, but when carried out by a person who has previously perpetrated serious assaults either outside or within the hospital, they convey a powerful threat. On occasion direct threats were explicitly made. These could be directed towards nurses or their families, and include descriptions of what the patient would do on release, threaten a formal complaint based on a false but credible allegation, violence, or even murder in the short term. All of these methods would be accompanied by the promise that any threat or burden would immediately disappear if the nurse would only comply with the patient's request.

Corrupting

This may involve tempting the nurse with the fascination of the forbidden, or direct corruption through escalating bribery, using money, drugs or other favours as payment. Unsurprisingly there is only one account of this in the interviews, and hopefully nurses succumbing to such offers would be rare. *I've been made aware of, of other staff who have felt that they're going along great guns, getting on well with people, with the individual patient, and may do something, or that person will push the boundary and it could be something as trivial as saying 'Could you get me something when you're out shopping, and I'll give you 20 fags' or whatever.*

Conditioning

This is an incremental erosion of the professional and objective nature of the staff–patient relationship. Comparison of the accounts of different nurses revealed a number of strategies used by patients to sway them through the development of special relationships:

Flattery The nurse becomes the recipient of praise about appearance, personal qualities or psychological skill. In offering help, gratitude is expressed, charm and niceness deployed, intimacy offered by the apparent sharing of things hidden or not normally spoken about (e.g. abuse or index offence personal histories).

Show of vulnerability   Inner pains and weaknesses are shared, keying into a desire to help and nurture, leading the nurse to consider the interaction deeply meaningful and productive, validating their role and self-image.

Sympathy   This is expressed for the nurse's difficulties in dealing with the management of other patients' behaviour, and for their position within the team. Areas of tension between the nurse and other team members, disciplines or their managers are identified and sympathized with.

Protection   Overt protection from other patients may be offered, and when the nurse gets into difficulties with another patient they will be defended, verbally or physically, generating a sense of indebtedness.

Humour   Use of a joking manner, making fun of themselves and others, in order to make any interaction enjoyable.

Parity demand   Mutuality is required as a moral obligation, forceful arguments are made that trust requires trust, risks should be shared, criticism should be accepted in both directions, respect should operate both ways, and that surely the nurse is not perfect and must have personal psychological problems. This may be coupled with gentle speculation on what these might be, based on careful daily observation, or identification of the problems the nurse has in relating to them. Alternatively, revelation of personal information may be required from the nurse as the price for continued self-revelation by the patient. Sometimes this may culminate in a reversal of the therapy, with the patient assisting the nurse with his psychological difficulties.

Incremental erosion of boundaries   Gradually increasing requests for special favours, starting with minor items, and copiously rewarded on each occasion.

Assertion of PD perspective   Eloquence in expressing their view of the world, themselves as victims within it, and the attribution of responsibility for their predicament onto others. The view is superficially plausible, permeates all interactions and is argued with great skill. It may be extended to incorporate the nurse as a fellow victim in a hostile world, cementing the alliance and friendship. The nurse's social reality may then shift from that shared in common with the everyday world, towards that of the patient's distorted PD perspective. Perversely, attaining the PD view of the world appears to be equivalent to gaining insight into the inner motivations of others, the social and psychological ghosts behind the sometimes mystifying world of interpersonal activities and relations.

Vacillation   Once the relationship has been established, further momentum is gained by alternating between positive and negative feedback. Movement towards fulfilling needs is rewarded by praise; failure to deliver is punished by disappointment and guilt induction.

When nurses talked about maintaining their 'boundaries' this could refer to the avoidance of conditioning relationships with patients. Sometimes the word 'boundary' was just used as a synonym for 'rule', and at other times it was used to refer to the distinctions between being a professional nurse and being a friend to patients: here the demarcations would be about self-disclosure, or the acceptance of gifts. However on yet other occasions they were using the term in the sense of 'ego boundary'. The picture of conditioning portrayed in this way is of patients encroaching upon the nurse's personal integrity, psychologically invading and colonizing the nurse with their own wishes, desires, intentions and perceptions. Thus talk about 'crossing boundaries' or 'maintaining boundaries' was, for staff, a powerfully metaphorical picture of the danger presented by conditioning relationships. Such relationships can be developed gradually, and they are not easy for staff to distinguish from genuinely therapeutic relationships. They may feed the conscious and unconscious needs of staff, and thus represent a powerful temptation. If not identified at an early stage, such relationships can result in the progressive erosion of security and other rules in favour of the patient. If the nurse and patient possess compatible sexualities, there is the danger that a romantic relationship can develop.

Capitalizing

This involves exploitation of available systems by the patient to the fullest possible extent using lies and deception. Examples given by the nurses and further described below are the use PD patients make of complaints and legal systems, the Mental Health Act and its code of practice, Patients' Councils, Advocacy Services, etc. These systems are available alternative avenues to authority and control, and can be used as leverage over the nursing hierarchy and nurses' control over the ward. *I've, patients who've been involved in the patients council, I've known patients there who are diagnosed as personality disorder and have tried to use the influence of being in the patients council, to, to influence nursing decisions on the ward to their advantage, not to the advantage of the ward or other patients but to their advantage.*

Conning

This includes exploiting the ignorance, lack of knowledge, or basic presumption of trustworthiness, mainly of new nurses but also of the unskilled, poor performers, the naïve and the unsuspicious. It may also involve the development of trust and commitment, to be exploited at a later date when privileges are given. Examples of the latter, given in the interviews, are of patients who say all the right things and pretend to make therapeutic progress, only to re-offend on discharge, or of patients who gain trust in order to get leave, and then abscond. *But what we've got to watch here with PD patients, is they can be manipulative, and they can say that they're doing, they're getting better, and they can conform to all the treatments they're having and yet they're not, they're only doing it for their own benefit. To get out of this place. And, and when they've been discharged, they've re-offended.*

Dividing

This can be interpreted as the creation of antagonism and conflict between others by the telling of lies, falsehoods or exaggerations of different sorts to different parties. Commonly called 'splitting the team', conflicts can be induced between nurses on the ward team itself, or between nurses and their managers, or between lower and higher grades of ward nursing staff (e.g. refusing to accept instructions from junior staff), or between male and female staff, or between the different psychiatric professions in the multi-disciplinary team. *They will try to manipulate, play one against the other, which they are expert at because they have been doing that for far longer than anyone can imagine, so here we have added problems.*

There was no relationship between the types of manipulation mentioned by nurses during the interview, and their overall attitude to PD. However, PD unit nurses had more to say about manipulation and were more likely to give descriptions of the various types.

The manipulation hexagon

The six-fold taxonomy of manipulation described above is somewhat idealized. Any one manipulative goal decided upon by a patient may require the use of a combination of methods, which may themselves overlap at one and the same time. This is depicted in Figure 3.1 by arranging the six types around the linked corners of a hexagon.

Instrumental manipulation appears transparent in motivation. It is deployed in order to acquire objects that cannot easily be gained in any other way, e.g. extra cigarettes, desired food items, a television set, pornography, alcohol, drugs, escape, etc. To a degree, manipulation towards these ends is normal within an institutional–prison environment. The attempted exploitation of staff within such an environment is also normal, as they are seen as the face of the authorities who keep the inmates captive against their will. The interviewed nurses gave many examples of this type of manipulation, e.g. a patient secures a television by taking advantage of a mentally ill patient, or attempts to bully a member of staff into bringing in drugs.

Interpersonal manipulation must be suspected when the goals are absent, obscure, bizarre, trivial, extreme or the strategy is so self-defeating that the

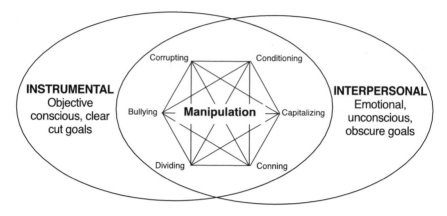

Figure 3.1 The manipulation hexagon.

end in view must have been other than the superficially obvious. Nurses described patients who manipulated situations 'not for positive gain' but simply because they could, or because they found it or the consequences in some way entertaining. The purpose the behaviour serves thus requires an alternative explanation, such as: an expression of the desire to dominate and acquire feelings of self worth; to be intimate with the person manipulated in order to obtain positive regard; an expression of anger/rage in response to real or supposed slight; to obtain recognition as a real human being; an acting out of inner emotional chaos. These explanations are derived from psychoanalysis (particularly the object relations school) and cognitive-behaviour therapy.

Instrumental and interpersonal manipulation are not mutually exclusive, and any one strategy may be serving both purposes for the patient at the same time. Both may be seen as originating in childhood. Instrumental manipulation would appear to be learned from the example of others and from the result of innate childhood problem-solving. The amorality of instru-mental manipulation may also be learned from a hostile and unloving family environment. Interpersonal manipulation, however, is the expression of a fundamentally flawed emotional outlook upon life and others, possibly originating from abuse or emotional deprivation.

Clever, intelligent and insightful

Implicit in the concept of manipulation is the idea that PD patients plan their devious schemes. The text of the interviews was therefore investigated for any references to plotting, planning, scheming or their synonyms. Identification of this aspect of PD behaviour, as with manipulation in general, was not related to overall attitude to PD. Most linked plotting to specific behaviours:

assaults on staff, escapes and hostage-taking. Occasions on which PD patients had made complex plans to assault staff, or even to murder them, were described. These plans included the use of other patients and events as distractions, and the preparation and concealment of weapons. Similar stories of the propensity of PD patients to plan escapes were related. Two accounts of patients planning to take staff as hostages were recounted, and in one of these the patient had sharpened a locker key on brickwork in order to use it as a weapon.

Another concept frequently associated by nurses with manipulative behaviour was that of intelligence. A text search of the interviews was therefore completed on the words clever/intelligent and their synonyms. A significant number of nurses asserted that PD patients were in some way intelligent or clever. For some, this meant being able to converse in a straightforward way that was beyond the ability of acutely psychotic patients; while for others it meant that the patients were educated or academic in certain respects. However, the largest number reported that PD patients were clever in the sense of being practiced, skilled, meticulous, and thoughtful in the way they manipulated others. There was no relationship between seeing PD patients as clever, skilled and crafty in deception, and overall attitude to PD.

When the nurses claimed that PD patients were intelligent, they were primarily drawing attention to their subtlety and craftiness, how they worked to hidden goals, and executed devious, complex plans with skill and a deft touch. These manipulative strategies would be carried out sequentially, over a long period of time, without being obvious and were seldom discovered before their fruition. Another aspect of PD intelligence was, in the eyes of the nurses, being clever at acting a role, carrying out a deception, lying effectively and convincingly over a long period of time without being found out. Simulating response to therapy in order to give a show of being fit for discharge was a particular example.

Some nurses described losing arguments with PD patients in relation to confrontations over hospital rules, even being driven to doubt themselves by the forcefulness and persistence of the attack. Others remarked upon the cleverness and duplicity displayed in garnering information about nurses for use in future manipulation. Lastly, some nurses observed a special cleverness in conditioning strategies, where the nurse's perspective is slowly and incrementally eroded to the point of becoming a tool in the hands of the patient.

Cleverness in this sense is not about IQ or academic intelligence, but about skilled deception. To the person who never contemplates the possibility of using manipulation, or who is basically honest, such behaviour would be difficult to carry out and maintain. Thus the manipulative strategies of PD patients are at first hard to identify or see, and appear to be executed with skill and precision. However, this seems to be more an issue of knowledge and practice, rather than of native intellectual talent.

The targets of manipulative strategies

Respondents gave a large number of examples as to how PD patients manipulate the nursing staff. It was clear from the interviews that it is experience of this type of behaviour that leads nurses to feel vulnerable and cautious when dealing with PD patients. One nurse gave an example of a new patient, recently admitted to the ward, who was very nice, and helpful towards the staff by telling them what other patients were doing and saying. The staff subsequently discovered that it was 'all a pack of lies', but at the time it seemed so genuine that the information conveyed about other patients was recorded in their files. It was the consistency and regularity of patients' manipulation that led another nurse to declare as a truism 'if he's breathing he's lying'.

The nursing staff were not alone in their vulnerability to manipulation. Other patients were also victims. A drawback to mixing PD and other patients on conventional wards was identified by some nurses, in that the PD patients were able to manipulate the mentally ill (i.e. psychotic) through greater social skills and virtuosity in using them. PD patients also sought to exploit and manipulate each other. The informal hierarchy that develops (and can be problematic for nurses to contain) is described in more detail below.

Solicitors were sometimes seen to be manipulated by PD patients. Examples given by the nurses were of their bringing banned items in or out of the hospital (e.g. tape recorders, mail, phone cards); giving time, input, and support; believing patients' tales without discussion with the nurses. All the examples given by nurses of doctors being manipulated related to medication and dosages. The nurses asserted that patients could sometimes get the medication they desired through demands or via presenting suitable symptoms to the medical staff. Relatives and friends were also perceived to be potential victims of patient manipulation, specifically with reference to the bringing of forbidden items into the hospital (e.g. illicit drugs). PD patients were seen to exploit the fear and concerns of managers by wielding influence outside the hospital (a high-profile patient might contact MPs and the media); by employing the managers' lack of awareness of their manipulative strategies to open gaps in procedures and policy that allow further exploitation; and by identifying, highlighting, exaggerating, or presenting in a twisted manner the deficits of individual staff, prompting management intervention.

Nurses talked about 'the system' being manipulated by patients, and this meant different things in different contexts. It was possible to identify at least three systems that, in the consideration of nurses, were abused by PD patients through manipulation: the legal system, the treatment system, and the complaints system. PD patients were perceived by some nurses as manipulating the legal system in order to obtain a transfer from the less desirable prison to the more pleasant environment of the hospital. In order to do so, they feigned symptoms of disruptive mental illness. Patients referred to this as being 'nutted off'. *Many patients have talked to me about behaviours they have displayed say in prison, and the terms that they use is 'I was facing a long stretch so I decided to get nutted off so that the life will be easier.'* Patients could also try to manipulate their way out of hospital by engaging in therapy purely to show that they had made an effort, or deliberately acting as if they were 'better', when they were not. This could result in some disenchantment for nurses who had made an emotional investment in the therapeutic process and had come to believe that they had seen patients progress, only to discover that they had been deliberately misled. There was a perception among some nurses that PD patients manipulated the complaints system, using it either to threaten staff and exert pressure on them, or to have unpopular staff suspended or moved to other areas of the hospital. This is discussed in more detail below. The total sum of the manipulative behaviour of patients, and its degree of success, led some nurses to conclude that PD patients were more powerful than staff, or were, in effect, 'running the hospital'.

Self-mutilation and disfigurement

Self-harm is particularly common among female PD patients, and can be frequent and severe. Nurses described patients who inserted pens or wires into themselves, cut themselves with broken crockery or glass creating large wounds, poking things in their eyes, swallowing batteries and other items or burning themselves with cigarettes. Repeated episodes over a long period could result in severe scarring and deformity, with limbs becoming 'a mass of scar tissue', or burns to 'every part' of the body.

Such behaviour was seen by some to be manipulative, with one nurse recollecting a patient who had said 'I've got to have it sorted now otherwise I'm going to cut myself or I'm going to overdose'. The same nurse then gave an example of a patient, who, when asked to wait to see a qualified nurse, broke a CD and cut herself with it. Other examples given were of patients who cut themselves to get off the ward and visit the general hospital, or to avoid an unwanted ward transfer. The words 'attention seeking' were used in a similar fashion, with cutting being seen as a deceitful way to obtain one-to-one interaction with nurses on demand, via the required treatment or the subsequent special observation by nurses to prevent further episodes. A few nurses commented on how angry and frustrated repeated cutting could make them. They also reported feeling distressed, traumatized and stressed by the sheer 'blood and gore' awful things they had to deal with, and by the high level of the patients' distressing emotions.

Exhibitions and displays of weakness or distress can be perceived as tyrannical. A common emotional response to such behaviour is to feel dominated, controlled by the need or the implied demand to be charitable, caring and concerned. A sense of coercion is induced via the normative obligation to set aside personal needs and desires to minister to distressed individuals, or make allowances for their weaknesses. Such feelings typically arise when the suffering person is deemed to be unreasonable, requesting more care than normal, or possibly acting or exaggerating. It is in these circumstances that nurses feel levered on the fulcrum of their everyday morality, or the demands of their moral nursing commitments. Under the duress of this perceived coercion, nurses are liable to call behaviour like this 'manipulative', and view it as a form of 'bullying'. Thus, in remarkably different settings (but having the same common denominator), nurses can feel manipulated by their patients. One of these scenarios is, as we have seen, the occurrence of self-injury by patients, to which nurses can feel compelled to give care and attention.

Not all nurses perceived deliberate self-harm in these terms. Far more saw it as a response to, or expression of, overwhelming negative emotions such as anger, guilt, shame, remorse, disappointment, worthlessness, etc. Others saw it as a tension-relieving device, a way of releasing internal anxiety in a strangely satisfying way. Some nurses indicated that patients could learn to deal with their emotions through self-harm, and that patients copied each other through contact and exposure in hospitals and prisons. Some regarded cutting as directly parallel to violence, with women more likely to take the former route of expression, and men the latter. However in a particularly illuminating comment, one nurse said that although she had no difficulty intellectually in understanding cutting as emotional expression, it was still difficult to accept it and treat the patient accordingly. This could be understood to mean that there are natural responses to self-injury (e.g. horror, anger, frustration) that are not easy to contain or ignore, and contaminate interactions with patients.

Aggression and violence

Many forms of violence are enacted by patients within the hospital. Verbal abuse and harassment can be frequent or continuous. Although this might seem trivial, several nurses remarked that this was harder to tolerate than actual physical violence, which was at least over and done with quickly. These verbal attacks can be personalized, and focus on the perceived psychological weaknesses of the staff member against whom they are directed. Sometimes they indicate rising tension and the possibility of a more serious attack, creating further stress on the nurse who is trying to handle and de-escalate the incident. Nurses described having to sit with disturbed patients for many hours while being the subject of the most vile abuse: *what they're not going to do to you, and what they are going to do to you, you know and you've got your mother and father you know – you're everything you know, you're horrible.* Another nurse described being targeted by a patient for three days of 'non-stop comments, bickering, back biting and arguing'.

Non-verbal intimidation and threats also occur. Nurses may be followed around in a hostile and threatening manner by a particular patient, or have to cope with threatening eye contact or continuously demanding behaviour that seeks to elicit a hostile response. Given that this is coming from patients who have committed serious and violent crimes, it can be highly stressful for nurses. *I have come across stares and intimidation, trying to intimidate you with their eyes. Movement, walk too close to you, or don't keep away when you're walking, challenging you for, more or less, psychological, try to, you know challenging you psychological. Looking at you straight in your eyes and – who's going to stop looking first.* Direct challenges and threats are common. These threats can include death, rape, taking the nurse hostage, and the making of serious (but fabricated) complaints. Patients occasionally threaten nurses' families and children, saying what they will do on release from the hospital, and such threats can be particularly intimidating. As a result, nurses tend to be very secretive about personal information that would allow patients some form of leverage. *There was an incident involving a couple of guys, where they did threaten me . . . It was amazing the way the incident arose, to see them change from two totally nice guys, to these two who were out to kill me . . . And they just kind of turned on me all of a sudden. . . . They were both there saying – all kinds of verbal threats. Yeah, it was a bit spooky.*

The actual physical violence that can occur within the hospital can be extremely serious and involve the use of weapons. Nurses mentioned that patients had wielded hot chip pan oil, boiling milk, knives, infected body fluids, boiling water, chair legs, pieces of glass, metal cooking implements, a razor blade, a TV aerial, a carving knife, flaming aerosols, a snooker cue, a table, and had also made attempts at poisoning, strangling, biting, head butting, and pushing a spoon into an ear. Such attacks are not always successful, but nurses do get injured, sometimes seriously. Nursing injuries enumerated included: cut mouth requiring stitches; broken cheek-bone; scalding of the neck and back; near strangulation; throat cut requiring surgery; broken nose; broken thumb; black eyes; head injury from being clubbed; fractured ribs, neck problems and tinnitus; knife slashes; knee strikes to the face; and being knocked unconscious. Following the more severe incidents injured nurses might be off duty for weeks, months, or over a year. Some nurses retire early or leave the service as a direct consequence of these attacks, and those who stay can suffer a severe loss of confidence and psychological ability to do the job.

Of particular concern to nurses were the carefully planned attacks of some PD patients, some of whom are capable of setting up a situation, in co-operation with other patients, to isolate and attempt to kill a member of staff. Several accounts of such actions were related in the interviews. Hostage-taking was also a concern: a small number had been taken hostage by a patient, or staff had managed to discover that such plans were afoot and prevented them from reaching fruition. Attacks are not always directed at the nurses; in many cases the patients attack each other, and nurses then become involved as they seek to contain the incident. Some of these attacks between patients are so severe that they can result in permanent disability or the death of the victim, and may require police investigation and prosecution. However, the nurses did not relate any attack on a staff member that resulted in prosecution. A further concern and worry for nurses was the possibility that, having physically restrained a patient, the patient would then make a complaint of assault. The result was often an investigation into the nurse's behaviour, not that of the patient.

Two-thirds of the nurses interviewed had been attacked or seriously threatened by a PD patient during the course of their career. Nurses had a pragmatic view of violence, and offered much more detailed thought about its immediate triggers than the long-term causes. 'Triggers' are more under the nurses' control, and are situations that nurses can be aware of and utilize in order to predict, prevent or contain aggression. Three items, discussed below, were particularly prominent in the list of aggression triggers that were identified.

Saying 'no'

This was the most frequently mentioned trigger to patient violence. It might mean specifically refusing a patient's request, but also means more broadly any action taken to limit or set constraints upon a patient's freedom of action. This can result in complete loss of temper on the patient's part, involve physical violence, or prompt verbal abuse or threats of imminent violence. Some nurses perceive this as intimidation or bullying – an attempt by patients to dominate them. *So basically it was, his reaction, their reaction, violence, and that was how he used to, hopefully achieve his ends.* Others saw it more simply as a complete loss of self-control generated by comparatively trivial frustration. *The member of staff working in the shop realized and said to him, 'No, you can't have a Mars bar because you are a Diabetic aren't you?' And he went – berserk I think's the word. Wrecked the shop – and he was restrained on the floor.* Being predictably faced with this type of behaviour means that nurses can be reluctant to place limitations on patients, especially when they know that saying 'No', even over trivial matters, can have serious consequences: *And they had made a plan to kill, 'cos they didn't like him, and felt he was too strict and you know.* Most persevere because they know it to be a necessary part of the role, one nurse referring to it as 'the art of confrontation'. Others will, on occasion, give way, simply to save trouble. *It makes you wary of them, it makes you wary of what you do when you are working with them. Sometimes when you should be not stricter but more upfront, you think, oh I am not going to say that, I am not going to say 'No you can't have that' because it won't be worth the trouble . . . why should I put my neck on the chopping block, you know. So sometimes I will just let it go if it is just minor.*

Nurse manner or attitude

Although hedged with provisos, and without exculpating the patient, some nurses made the point that the nurse-victim's manner or attitude could itself contribute to the triggering of violence. For some, this was about failure to explain decisions or refusals; for others it was about inappropriate responses by the nurse, or critical comments, or body language that could be interpreted as hostile. *I've been threatened but that was to do with me folding my arms basically. I suppose obviously he thought it was a hostile act basically.* One nurse made the point that it was about how the patients were spoken to, and that some staff were repeatedly victims because of their manner. *I think a lot of this has got to do with negative attitude on the part of the staff as well. If you have a negative attitude towards that person, if you approach that person as though he is just a nonce or he is a person who is not capable of doing something, then he will more than likely show his aggression more.* Another saw it as a matter of having an easy-going personality, and the ability to get on with people. *I think you can go in sometimes and have an air of aggression about you or an air of silence and people are wary of you and that can create barriers. It can create the opposite, the friction where you can bring on assault or attack or abuse, from your own personality towards people.*

Relatives

Several nurses mentioned violence as being triggered by relatives' visits. As all interviewees were asked about the effects of relatives' visits, the frequency of these comments may simply reflect the fact that this question was asked. Nevertheless, those nurses who did comment on this issue gave examples showing how the frustrations of visits, or anger expressed during them, could overflow onto the ward after the visit had taken place. It is also clear that, through interaction with the patients or their relatives, nurses can become embroiled or implicated in family dynamics that carry strong emotional reactions. These dynamics can then elicit violence from the patient. *Came back from the visit, was frightened and very frustrated that his parents were going to try and get him out, walked round the ward, tried to find out who was in charge of the ward, . . . asked one of the nurses who was on duty tonight, er, did you, are you in charge? He said yes and he beat seven bells of shit out of him, really, really bad attack put him off for six weeks.*

Effects of violence on nurses

Some nurses advanced the idea that attacks created negative attitudes to PD, but this was not supported by the findings of this study. Although 67 per cent of the sample had been attacked or seriously threatened by a PD patient, there was no significant correlation between this and overall attitude to

PD. The links between attitude and response to violent incidents were more complex than a simple correlation between being a victim and the possession of a negative attitude. The main emotional responses of nurses to a violent incident are given below.

Nurses were commonly angry following an attack, and that anger had a number of different forms and rationales. For some it was simply anger directed at the patient coupled with a natural desire for revenge: *I think sometimes it crosses your mind that there's an awful lot you'd like to do like hit back or whatever, but you can't because obviously, it's not your job to do that, it's not what you're here for, but it's normal isn't it?* For others, it was the contrast between the fact that the nurse had been trying to help the patient, and yet had still been assaulted, that accentuated the angry feelings. *I see the nursing staff trying to help them, so therefore when they do something like that I feel extremely let down and angry, that they would do something like that to one of us.* For yet others, it was the injustice of the assault, the fact that it was not justified by the trivial matter that triggered it, that led to angry feelings. Some nurses reported that they became angrier with PD patients following an assault, because they knew what they were doing and were more responsible than psychotic patients. *So, yes it was planned, well organized and it made me angry because he knew what he was doing and he showed no remorse. So, yes it makes me angry.* This anger cannot be expressed as the nurses know it is wrong and unprofessional to do so. Yet it is coupled by some to frustration at the fact that there is little in the way of sanctions or consequences for violent behaviour within the High Security Hospital system. That anger can also generalize to the managers for allowing a violence-provoking situation to develop or for policies that were perceived to put nurses at risk (e.g. patient access to boiling water), or to those who represented the patients' interests (e.g. Solicitors, Advocates, Mental Health Act Commissioners). There was no relationship between the expression of anger at attacks and overall attitude to PD, indicating that it is a normal response that does not have any enduring impact on nurses' general approach to patients. Anger about attacks did not therefore necessarily lead to the rejection of PD patients.

Many nurses admitted to feeling vulnerable, worried, anxious, frightened, threatened, intimidated, tense, on edge, and terrified during or following attacks. Those who mentioned this also saw it as a normal response to violent events. *When I talk about her now I get sweaty palms, that's how much she frightened me.* As with anger, there was no relationship between the expression of fear and overall attitude to PD, indicating the normality of the response and the fact that it does not necessarily lead to long-term feelings of vulnerability.

Other nurses reported being more security conscious and cautious following a violent incident. This was because they had been reminded in a particularly graphic way of what the patients were capable of doing. This implies that there is a natural process by which nurses become less cautious over time, perhaps driven by the establishment of good, productive working relationships with patients. Then the occurrence of violence comes as a shock, causing nurses to re-evaluate their situation. *Even more wary of the environment that I work in, because unfortunately when things go relatively smoothly, there is the possibility that you might have a tendency to forget where you are and the dangers that you are in. So immediately it makes you more aware of the environment that you're working in.* There was a correlation between voicing longer-term wariness following an attack, and overall negative attitude to PD. This suggests that, for some nurses, fear created during or following an attack becomes a sustained and enduring part of their approach to PD patients, whereas for the more positive nurses the fear is short lived. Perhaps some nurses have more unrealistic expectations about the behaviour of PD patients, and respond with a more acute 'let down', coupled with fear, when violence occurs, leading to a more enduring vulnerability and cynicism.

Some nurses state they are completely unaffected by the attacks of patients, that they have become hardened, or accept it as part of the job. This may be because, in the culture of the hospital, expressions of fear are prohibited and toughness is valued. *It makes you feel terrified, it can, I mean I was assaulted . . . actually knocked out, sent off duty, I was conscious when I went off duty, but I don't know. It took me a long time to actually get over that and I used to openly admit to people I was scared of coming back, I didn't feel confident and I think I used to horrify some people. Because you don't tell people that.* It may be that this prohibition helps nurses to overcome and hide their fear; on the other hand, it may inhibit them from working their way through it, and it certainly prevents them from receiving psychological support from the nursing team. The numbers of nurses saying they were unaffected is too small to discover any correlation with overall attitude. Another small group of nurses reported feeling stressed or depressed because of violence, either saying they felt 'down', or that following an incident the whole ward felt 'down', or that afterwards they went home feeling 'stressed out'.

Following an incident some nurses will ruminate about how they could have handled things differently to avoid the incident. In one sense this is helpful, because it turns any event into a learning process. In another sense nurses may get a feeling of guilt for an incident that could not have been avoided, and that in any case was really the responsibility of the perpetrator. *But when you get hit or find yourself in a position, you always look at the guilt on yourself. 'I should never have been in that position. I should never have been there, I should have been able to see, and I should have been aware of the possibility of it happening.'*

There are several factors that influence how nurses feel following an incident. The first emotional reactions, which are the most acute, tend to fade fairly quickly, with nurses able to resume their duties after a few days 'as if nothing has happened'. The more severe the attack and its consequences, the more acute and long-term is the emotional response. One notorious occasion, in which a nurse's throat had been cut in an attack by a patient, was mentioned by several nurses as resulting in feelings 'running high'. Lastly, feelings are more acute when the attack comes from a patient with whom the nurses felt they had a good relationship that was working therapeutically. In this context, a reaction of acute disappointment ensues, which is described in more detail in the chapter that follows. Nurses do sometimes leave the service after witnessing violence or being assaulted: *And she got attacked three times or four times within a two-year period, quite serious attacks, she got a broken nose, a broken thumb, four stitches in her lip, and then the last time she came home with a black eye and scratches all down her face. And since then she's, she's resigned, well she's took early retirement. Her confidence went really and she just, couldn't hack it anymore.*

Criticisms and complaints

Virtually all interviewees had something to say about the criticisms and complaints made by patients, underlining the importance of the topic to them. Although nurses were not specifically asked about whether they had been the subjects of formal complaints by PD patients, many spoke about this. Based on this interview survey, about one in six nurses have been in this position. This figure could be higher, as nurses may be reluctant to share this information. In addition, the figure does not include those nurses who resign due to stress and anger about the procedure, or those who are dismissed when complaints are upheld. Nurses who have been the subjects of complaints were very much less likely to support the notion that criticisms and complaints should be encouraged, and were more likely to have a negative overall attitude to PD patients. It is impossible to tell the direction in which these associations operate. Being subject to a complaint may generate negative attitudes, or negative attitudes might express themselves in behaviour that leads to complaints. The relationship might in fact be bidirectional – operating in both ways simultaneously.

Staff recognized that patients frequently had good cause and justifiable reasons for making complaints. Nurses acknowledge that service deficits exist, and appreciate that patients can become angry about them and eventually complain. These deficits can be such things as: lack of escorts to therapeutic activities; inequities in the sharing out of meals and other consumables; difficulties in accessing the hairdressers, etc. Occasionally they are about staff misconduct, or contested treatment decisions.

However, nurses also identified many less positive dynamics behind the making of complaints by patients. For example, nurses also attributed patient complaints to the desire to accumulate power and dominate through manipulative behaviour. Thus nurses relate how patients make false and malicious allegations, or threaten to do so, in order to coerce the nurse to give way and seriously bend or break rules. Patients are also perceived as making complaints in order to get nurses suspended or moved from the wards, and then to celebrate or boast about this when it occurs, using the accrued prestige to move up the informal patient hierarchy. Nurses describe this behaviour as 'getting you into trouble', 'dropping you in it', 'turning on you', and the complaints procedure itself is seen by some as 'administrative violence' and a 'weapon', or in other words an instrument of threat and domination. Thus PD patients are seen as a very powerful group within the hospital via their use of the complaints procedure: *It just seems to be they run, they run the management.*

Some complaints were seen as originating in problematic nurse–patient relationships. Examples were: a nurse expressing disrespect for a patient; a patient not liking a nurse or taking an instant dislike to one individual staff member; a patient being angered by a nurse refusing something; jealousy of a nurse's good relationship with another patient. Yet others were perceived to be an outcome of patient frustration with delays. However good the reason for a delay, PD patients can sometimes respond with a complaint when their requests are not immediately dealt with. The interviewees relate both formal and informal complaints that have resulted from asking patients to wait for a cup of tea, to have a letter posted, to get access to the telephone, or to have nurses' assistance in the search for a missing cup. Complaints of assault seem to be particularly common after a violent incident during which the patient is restrained, with this scenario being mentioned by nearly one in ten nurses: *Harms himself with a weapon, covers himself with excrement, patient, staff go in, kid gloves, handle it really well, you smacked me in the mouth. Complaint, suspension, bingo.* Lastly, engagement with the complaints process is seen by some nurses as a deliberate distraction from the real issues that face the patient, while others suggest that a complaint may represent a cry for help in another area.

Nurses' responses to criticisms and complaints could be strongly emotional. On these occasions nurses could feel betrayed, disappointed and let down by the patients whom they were trying to help and care for. In addition, their sense of control over events was threatened in an environment in which it was very important that they maintain control – for their own safety and that of their colleagues and the general public. Finally, if the complaint was about the nurse as an individual, then that person's livelihood and future career were threatened. These issues were reflected in the topics mentioned by nurses when talking about criticisms and complaints.

Nurses felt victimized, hurt, distressed, insulted and betrayed, as if a slur had been cast on their character, integrity and honesty. It was the contrast between their very real efforts to help patients and receiving a complaint that they found most painful: *Yeah people complain about all sorts of shit, and it's awful. You work really hard, really, really hard, you bend over backwards and . . . then you get a complaint through. You get a complaint that, that, that you were abusive that you attacked someone or it's nonsense.* 'Guilty until proven innocent' was a frequent comment, particularly in relation to how nurses believed their managers perceived them during the investigation of a complaint The formal complaints process is lengthy and extremely stressful for staff, who often felt that their livelihood was under threat (and hence the security of their families). Some responded to these circumstances by constant worry, losing weight, becoming sick; others simply left the hospital because they were unable to tolerate the uncertainties and threats of the process. *But we have had situations on here where, petty complaints have been made which have turned into, month and month long enquiries where, which have caused staff, and other patients to be fair, a lot of anxiety.*

Some nurses had difficulty fitting together what the patients complained about and the index offence that had brought them into hospital. To some nurses there seemed to be an essential contradiction between these two things. Where they expected sorrow, remorse and a certain amount of self-abnegation, they found instead patients who are keen to assert their own value and rights. Thus the expression of a complaint or criticism by a patient could arouse irritation in the nurse. *'Cos you know, you have committed a horrific offence, what do you expect? You are in a place to rehabilitate you and you are moaning the milk is warm.* One of the ways nurses reacted to a complaining patient was to increase the social distance between them and avoid contact with them, on the grounds that this reduced the things about them that the patient could complain about. Other nurses mentioned deploying a barrier of general wariness. Being the subject of a complaint made nurses conscious of their reputation within the hospital. They felt unfairly stigmatized, that their reputation as a nurse had been damaged. As one nurse put it, 'mud sticks', or, as another pointed out, regardless of the outcome it goes down on your record. *That's often talked about when there's staff suspended because of accusations a patient's made. And then obviously that staff and that patient get talked about.*

Whatever their motivation, patients do make malicious, false and sometimes trivial complaints. The NHS complaints procedure, coupled with the history of patient abuse in the High Security Hospitals, means that these complaints are dealt with carefully, fairly and objectively. However the formal complaints procedure can be very destructive, can cause much worry even among those who have only witnessed what it has done to others, and is costly in terms of management time, suspensions, illness and resignations at a time when nursing staff are a scarce resource. It is because of its very destructiveness that patients can use the threat of it to seek to coerce nurses into improper actions.

Mutual exploitation

The propensity of PD patients to establish an informal hierarchy, to manipulate each other or other mentally ill patients, was a management problem for nurses. Examples were given of patients arranging unfair deals for expensive items with payment rendered in cigarettes, or the holding of drugs or other illicit items. An uncontained patient hierarchy was said to result in:

- more fights and arguments;
- low ward patient morale;
- increased levels of tension fear, nervousness and insecurity among patients;
- deferential behaviour (cower, lie to support the dominant patient's complaints about staff, agreeing with that patient in his or her presence);
- giving gifts and treats, a form of investment in protection;
- copycat behaviour (e.g. cutting); leading others into trouble (strikes, rooftop protests).

It is difficult for the staff to know what is being planned, except indirectly through events not otherwise explicable, or through sensing an 'atmosphere', or through observing an increase in meetings between little groups of patients. The informal hierarchy of patients has its own descriptive vocabulary among nurses (and perhaps patients too). It is a 'ladder' or 'pecking order'. The dominant are called 'top dog' ('daddy of the day room' for female wards), 'wise boys' and 'rule the roost'. Patients who defer or are intimidated are called 'the lesser patients', 'weaker lads' and are 'bullied' or 'victimized'.

The methods patients use to seek to dominate each other were detailed in the interviews, and included:

- establishing a place in the hierarchy through intimidation, by threatening others outside of the view of nurses;
- using greater verbal fluency to win arguments and convince others to submit or comply;
- imposing their will on someone else by getting them to do something by devious means, thus demonstrating the possession of greater power; using manipulative skills, usually on more gullible or naïve patients;
- getting appointed to various committees or the patients' council, and using that position to seek satisfaction of their own goals;
- actual physical fights: injuring other persons, putting them in their place;
- cultivation of a reputation for being violent;
- monopolization of desired resources, e.g. telephone access, meals, etc;
- using the characteristics of other patients for scapegoating, e.g. the paedophiles who are looked down on by others;
- developing physical strength, as muscle mass and size gives status in the hierarchy;
- ganging up with other patients to dominate the ward.

Nurses have a number of methods for controlling and ameliorating the effects of the informal patient hierarchy. Indeed, preventing bullying from happening is one of the things that demonstrates that the nurses are effectively 'in charge'. They restrict the responsibilities and leadership given to patients, or do not allow the type that gives an opening to exploitation, or monitor and restrict it. Clear, open rules for conduct, which are consistently applied and uniformly imposed, prevent any one patient from gaining an advantage. Ensuring that the weaker patients can express their fears of certain patients openly at ward community meetings, and have them dealt with also restricts the scope for bullying. As a last resort, overly dominant patients are transferred to another ward, or a gang is split up by sending different members to different wards.

Summary

In short, psychiatric professionals who care for PD patients in forensic settings have a lot to cope with. They need to find positive ways to deal with their own emotional reactions to patients' past crimes and to their current behaviours. Those current behaviours include attempts by patients to manipulate the staff, using bullying, corrupting, conditioning, capitalizing, conning and dividing techniques. PD patients can be frightening and intimidating, crafty and clever in the way in which they seek to achieve their own ends. Those manipulative strategies can be directed against the staff, who then need to be on their guard, or against other patients, whom the staff need to protect from exploitation. On other occasions they can seek to harm themselves in ways that elicit strong feelings of repugnance and disgust. These patients can be so violent that they engender permanent stress, wariness and fear in the staff. At the same time they may utilize the administrative violence of the complaints process to put staff under yet more pressure.

Given this context it is not surprising that some nurses loathe working with PD patients, feel vulnerable when in their presence, reject them, feel that caring for them is futile, and are overwhelmed with exhaustion. However, although most nurses can recognize these feelings within themselves to some degree, there are many who have found a way to work with a positive attitude, enjoy caring for PD patients, feel secure in their presence and accepting towards them, having a sense of purpose and enthusiasm. How they do this will be described in the next chapter, and how the organization can support them in doing so will be the subject of Chapter 5.

4 Staying positive

The reasons why PD patients elicit negative reactions from those who care for them are now apparent. The bare facts of the survey have been provided with some context. The generally hopeless, pessimistic, angry attitudes of carers can be seen to originate in the difficult behaviours of PD patients. They bully, con, capitalize, divide, condition, and corrupt those around them. They make complaints over inconsequential or non-existent issues in order to manipulate the staff. They can be seriously violent over unpredictable and objectively trivial events, or may harm and disfigure themselves in ways that have an intense emotional impact on staff. If this were not enough, they also behave in the same way towards each other, provoking serious problems that the staff have to manage and contain. On top of this, the staff have to come to terms with the committed offences that have brought patients into hospital – offences that can be so grievous as to elicit feelings of disgust and abhorrence.

Yet there are some staff who manage in a more positive fashion than others. There are nurses who enjoy their work, feel safe, accepting towards patients, have a sense of purpose and who are enthusiastic. How they do this, and the impact that this has on them both inside and outside the hospital, are the topics explored in this and the following chapter. The methods positive staff used were revealed in the interviews, particularly during discussions about coming to terms with patients' index offences and how these were to be regarded. However, they were also displayed in talk about how the current ward behaviour of the patient was managed and construed, especially the disappointments the nurses underwent as part of trying to work therapeutically, and how they managed other emotion-eliciting events. Further factors that enabled staff to have a positive overall attitude were revealed when they spoke of their fundamental beliefs about the cause of PD, treatment of PD patients, and of their responsibility for their behaviour and offences. Finally, those with whom the nurses identified proved to be an unanticipated element in their ability to take a positive attitude to their work.

The powerful impact that working with PD patients in the High Security Hospitals had on staff should not be underestimated. For nurses who developed an overall negative attitude to PD patients, the impact could be psychologically and socially toxic. They were more likely to have conflict-based relationships with patients, eliciting more negative behaviour and responses from them and confirming their point of view. This was not the only impact, however, as these nurses took the effects outside the hospital, where they sometimes had a profound impact upon their personal lives.

Rejecting the terminology of evil

Nurses used a number of different cognitive strategies to cope with their natural reactions towards the actions of PD patients in their care. Most of these were based upon appeals to higher moral values or ideals, or were declarations of moral choices that nurses had taken in the past and still supported in the course of their work. These are presented below in no order of priority, as each morality or method received about the same degree of support, judged by the frequency with which they were described.

In these circumstances, nurses had recourse to the professional ideology of their discipline. Indeed much of the morality described in this section may be affiliated or associated with nursing. However, one element of this trans-cended nursing and related to the ideology of professionalism itself – affective neutrality. In this view professionals provide a service that is blind to the nature of the client. Thus solicitors provide legal advice, and nurses pro-vide nursing care. One interviewee referred to the terminology of evil as 'inappropriate terms' for the 'professional nurse–patient relationship', and another spoke of being 'totally blank and professional about it'. In short, what this seems to mean at a practical level is that when feelings of anger start to emerge towards patients for what they have done, nurses ignored or suppressed them on the grounds that their professional role of providing a caring service came first.

More specific to psychiatric nursing in the UK was an adherence to the value of accepting patients as individuals, and an appreciation that their mental health problems and personal history were unique to them. This ideology of individualized care is longstanding, and appears to be associated with a widespread acceptance of 'labelling theory' from sociology. Nurses descry the labelling and stigmatizing of patients, and have internalized the rejection of asylum care with its impersonal herding and processing of large numbers of patients. This same form of argument was used by some nurses as a reason to reject the terminology of evil: *I think it's, it's very easy for anybody with any kind of psychiatric illness to, to be labelled and I think it's something that all psychiatric nurses tend to work against, you know labels of kind of mad, or bad, or anything like that.* In other words, nurses who advanced this argument challenged themselves to get to know the patient as a person with a rich personal history and unique characteristics, instead of angrily and summarily rejecting them before becoming acquainted. Another nurse argued that they had learned during their training that they should accept 'people for what they are as individuals you know rather than just, carte blanche labelling somebody like that' and others argued that the task of nurses was to 'understand people' rather than call them names like 'monsters'.

Perhaps closer to the professionalism idea was a commitment to preventing the recurrence of crime. This provided a justification for ignoring emotional reactions to past offences, putting them to one side and engaging with the patient in order to make therapeutic progress: *All I know is that they've not done nice things, that's why they're here and part of my job is to make sure they don't do those not nice things again.* This method of coping can, of course, only be maintained as long as the nurse believes that treatment can work. Given the poor state of evidence for the efficacy of the treatment of PD, this stance may be more indicative of a leap of faith than anything else. For other nurses, the reason why anger (and the terminology of evil) was rejected was because all patients, even those who were PD, were considered mentally ill and therefore in need of nursing care. For other nurses the arguments in this area were more complex (see below), with distinctions drawn between patients suffering from psychosis, who were considered to be clearly ill and therefore not responsible for their behaviour, and PD patients who were not ill and were responsible. However, there were some nurses who argued that PD patients were ill and not responsible in a different way: *You're looking after people who don't know what they do. A mentally ill person doesn't know what he does. A PD patient doesn't know why, why he does what he does, and that's the difference. He probably know what he does, but he doesn't know why he does it.* For nurses who could argue this to themselves, the matter of the terminology of evil did not arise, as the personal agency and responsibility of patients was reduced or diminished. Another similar tactic was for nurses to remind themselves of the history of the abuse and suffering of the patients: *Some of their choice was not made for them because their early history, the deprivation, abuse they suffered wasn't their doing and what they are doing now is partly the result of what happened then. So I don't think those words are appropriate.* When patients apparently have no history of being abused, they are more likely to be considered evil or monstrous.

Some nurses fended off anger and the terminology of evil by reminding themselves that PD patients were still 'human beings': *There's certainly people that are hard to get at but it doesn't rule them out of the human race you know, we've all got a life to live no matter what way people tend to go.* It is unclear what exactly the nurses meant by this reply and others like it. Which characteristics of the patients were they internally recalling that justified their judging PD patients as 'human beings'? Why were they able to do this when others looked at the index offences and had no doubt that the PD patients had lost their entitlement to being regarded as full members of the human race? Perhaps there was nothing more here than an innate sensitivity or emotional reaction that provides this justification, and expression of compassion and pity: *At the end of the day they're human beings and they need looking after. I can agree with the statement of monster and evil but part of me says yes, at the end of the day, you know they're there and they do need looking after kind of thing. A lot of them don't think they need looking after but they do.* On the other hand, in the context of nurses' other statements about professional commitments to patients, plus their refusal to label them and write them off as 'evil', this stress on the humanity of patients probably links with personally held schemes of moral values on universal human equality and human rights.

A number of nurses indicated that they had tried to draw a distinction between PD patients' behaviour, which could be seen as evil and monstrous, and the patients themselves, who were not. They argued that although 'the acts' were evil, the patients could not be so described. Again, what this seemed to mean in practice was that nurses could put the negatively judged behaviour to one side, ignore it, and get on with developing a positive relationship with the patients. Thus they were able to satisfy their need to morally condemn patient behaviour, yet also follow their moral ideal of providing care and therapy. *One patient asked me if you know 'I bet you think I'm bad really don't you?' And I says 'No, what you did was bad but that doesn't make you bad and I want you to help by avoiding doing that in the future.'*

Such coping methods are mentioned very significantly more often by those with an overall positive attitude to PD, demonstrating that these are some of the means by which positive nurses achieve and maintain their feelings of enjoyment in the work, sense of security, acceptance of patients, sense of purpose and their enthusiasm.

Handling reading the case notes

Reading the case notes brought nurses face to face with the reality of what patients had done, and as such could arouse powerful feelings of anger, sadness, fear, incomprehension and disgust. The main way nurses had of dealing with the thoughts, preoccupations and emotions triggered by the index offence was by simply not thinking about it. This was variously articulated as: 'not dwelling on it', 'blocking it out', 'putting it at the back of your mind', 'cutting it out', 'put it out of mind', 'put on a different hat', 'cut yourself off', 'don't think about it', 'concentrate on other things', 'detach yourself', 'desensitize', 'put it onto the side', 'switch off', 'neutralize yourself', 'forget about it', 'ignore it', 'leave it on the back burner', 'put it behind you'. Others expressed it as a total separation between their work and home, with the transition being marked by coming through the perimeter gates and picking up the security keys when coming on duty. This seems to be almost a ritual that helps nurses to keep the boundary between their normal everyday reactions and feelings, and their professional selves. *You hang your mentality up when you come in and pick your keys up, and when you're going out, you leave work with your keys and you should never ever mix the two.* Some nurses questioned whether this was a healthy mechanism, but did not reach any certain answer, on the one hand considering that, regardless of any attempt to suppress feelings, these would have an effect at the end of the day, but on the other almost admiring the efficiency and totality with which it could be done There was no relationship between this widely used mechanism of suppression or dissociation, and overall attitude to PD. It remains a curious and unanswered question as to where these suppressed emotions (presumably those detailed above: anger, sadness, revulsion, fear) go, and whether they are expressed elsewhere or in disguised forms. It is also open to question whether nurses who keep their emotional responses under such tight control are actually able to discuss the patients' index offences with them in a therapeutic way, or whether, because they block thoughts about the index offence, they cease to assess properly the risks posed by the patient.

An allied method of dealing with the emotional consequences of reading case notes was not to read case notes, or only read them selectively. Those nurses who avoided reading the case notes at all preferred to gain information about the index offence and the dangers presented by patients from other nurses who did. By this means they distanced themselves from direct accounts of the index offence. Others read the case notes selectively, just enough to know the basics about the patients without being emotionally affected. *I try never to read, apart from that which I need to make sure that I'm safe and my, and the staff are safe.* Although this strategy was not associated with an overall negative attitude to PD, it must be questioned whether nurses who used it were able to do any therapeutic work with patients around their offending behaviour. Presumably, just as they blocked the details from their reading, these nurses similarly did not allow the topic to enter conversations with patients.

Although suppression of feelings and responses was common in both positive and negative nurses, the rationales given for it were different. One particular rationale for suppression was strongly associated with an overall negative attitude to PD. Nurses who loathed their work, felt insecure, rejecting of patients, felt their care was a waste of time and drained them of energy, were more likely to suppress their feelings about patients' index offences as a matter of necessity. They said that unless they cut themselves off from such feelings, they 'can't do their job', 'couldn't work here', 'would be too depressed to work', 'couldn't do therapy', 'it would drive me mad', or 'would have a nervous breakdown'. This position may be termed suppression to survive. In their comments, nurses gave the impression or sense that they were working against their natural grain and were denying some essential and valued part of themselves as human beings. *No, I think, most people have developed some way of detaching themselves from or certainly detaching the patient from the crime. Otherwise I don't think most human beings could work in this sort of environment.*

In this context a small number of staff spoke about avoiding patients as a means of containing reactions to their crimes. That this is not a desirable or acceptable way to deal with the emotions aroused by the index offence is reflected in the fact that nurses reported observing this in others to a far higher degree than admitting that they did this themselves. The self-reports acknowledge a certain psychological withdrawal from patients – a degree of distance that would not otherwise have been present, but a sense that awareness of the crime was always present in the background of any inter-action with the patient. So interviewees spoke of difficulty in talking to a patient 'without either feeling or showing some disgust at what they have done'. Reports about other nurses are more explicit, saying that those who can't accept serious crimes 'find it difficult to relate to the patient' and 'tend to have little to do with them'. *Well most of them they read the case notes, the index offence and from them they'll take a certain dislike, and whatever comes from them they'll say, 'well go away I don't want to know'.* Other respondents talked about nurses who had asked to move ward for a period in order to make the emotional adjustment to working with a certain patient, or nurses who did not engage in certain types of group therapy where index offence related material is likely to be discussed. What the patients got from nurses who cannot wholly contain their emotional response was nothing beyond 'the normal duties of care', a refusal to do anything extra for them, and nurses who interacted in an 'offhand manner'. To a degree, nurses under-stood each other's difficulties in this area, and would support each other by allocating patient care to facilitate a degree of avoidance, or would verbally support and encourage each other. The ultimate form of avoidance was for nurses to leave the High Security Hospital service, and eight examples of this were given by interviewees. *The nurse who started with me, she only lasted for three weeks and left. It was because of partly of case notes and this thing of saying how am I going to speak to this person when I know what he has done.* Although it seems likely that avoidance is related to overall nega-tive attitude to PD, the small numbers of self-reports make this impossible to assess statistically.

A number of self-management methods were mentioned in connection with reading the case notes and dealing with feelings about the index offence that, when grouped together, show an association with an overall positive attitude to PD. These are very similar to those methods by which nurses avoid thinking of patients as bad, evil or monstrous. The identical findings here strengthen the case that these are important psychological mechanisms, via which nurses contain their own emotions and make a positive adjustment to the issues involved in caring for PD patients who have committed serious and extreme offences.

A significant number of nurses spoke of being professional in their approach to patients, some of them connecting this to being nurses and the ideal of the profession. *I came into this job, I came into this job with my eyes open, I became a nurse and part of the talent of that is that I, apart of my code of conduct suggests that I have to deal, that I have to do the best for people.* These nurses saw themselves as having a positive role in the treatment of patients that made it possible to allow themselves to set to one side their natural feelings about the index offences, and talked about this as 'going into professional mode'. They were 'here for the patient', their overarching purpose was to 'empathize with them' and 'help them', and this was why they had chosen to work in the hospital. Their affiliation to the caring ideology of nursing assisted them in keeping and maintaining this position, staying objective rather than being overcome by their own emotional responses. *You've got a professional job to do, and we're nurses not prison officers, so we're here to find out, assess them and find out their problems and their backgrounds.* It is not that these nurses did not have normal emotional responses to patients' actions – they did and they were well able to articulate these, but, having had those emotional responses, they were able to put them away for the sake of achieving something better and more meaningful. *And it's like you, I understand that I work here and it's a case of balancing that and recognizing yes they do make me feel like this but I'm here to do a job, I've chosen to work here. And I will be part of the treatment team. It's almost a contradiction in terms of feeling, that's how I feel anyway. As soon as I walk through those gates, it's weird.* The issue of choice was mentioned by many nurses in connection with being a professional in this environment, and seemed to be an important component of being able to use this self-management method. Those who had not thought about these issues prior to becoming a nurse or before coming to work in the High Security Hospitals, and had not consciously made this decision, may not have been as able to make this positive adjustment to their role.

Concentrating attention on the person as he or she is now was another means by which nurses kept their emotional reactions under control. As an alternative to thinking about the past and the index offence, these nurses sought to concentrate on the person's current behaviour and the nurse's current relationship with that patient. They expressed this as 'the patient is the first priority', 'treat them on how they present', 'taking them at face value', 'seeing the person as opposed to the offence', 'look at the whole person, not just the index offence', 'get to know them as they are now', 'work with what I see', or 'treat them on how they respond now'. Interspersed were comments about patients being 'individuals' that resonate with what nurses had to say about the ideology of individualized care, and the anti-labelling perspective previously described. *Take them as you find them, don't put onto them everything in the case notes. Deal with them as they are today, is my other little whim.* Using this method is not without problems, and some nurses recognized this by mentioning that, for the sake of safety, they had to know about the index offence and not forget it completely. In addition, concentrating on individuals as they are now must pose some risk of being taken in and 'conned' or 'conditioned' by the well-known charm, niceness and manipulative ability of PD patients.

Keeping one's attention on the individuals as they are now could also be assisted, not by ignoring or avoiding reading the case notes, but by first making sure that the patients were known human beings. Nurses did this by meeting the patients first, getting to know them as persons, before finding out about their index offences or reading case notes. In this way it would appear that they were better able to balance the reality of each patient as an individual human being against a knowledge of what had been done. Some were very confident that this was a productive way of moving forward and meeting new patients, and recommended this as a course of action for all nurses. *There was one nurse here who, who taught me something very important really which was to actually meet with the individual and to get to know the individual first before reading their case notes. And what I find with doing that is that it's very, or it's easier then to put into perspective their past psychiatric history or offending history, when you actually know the person for who they are today.*

Another way nurses had of interpreting the meaning of their role within the hospital was by contributing to the prevention of further crimes. By being part of the team that was treating patients, they saw themselves as making it less likely that the terrible events that had happened would recur when the patients were discharged. This ideology gave them a rationale and justification for not thinking about the index offence or the hurt it had caused to others, with one nurse saying that she could not 'change what they have done in the past' but may be able to 'prevent them damaging further in the future'. Being able to hold this position is dependent on the nurses' belief that patients are treatable, and that they, as nurses, have a meaningful role and contribution to make to that treatment. This implies that it is important for nurses to have a valued role in the treatment programme of patients, and that to be excluded from such a role would contribute to the development of negative attitudes.

A small group of nurses stated an adherence to the value of 'non-judgementalism' that helped them to set aside their feelings towards patients. This avoidance of judging patients derives from Carl Rogers' client-centred therapy, where it is a core value and method of doing psychotherapy. The reference to non-judgementalism by nurses bears witness that Rogerian psychotherapy is popular and well known among UK psychiatric nurses, even if it is not necessarily practised in any pure form, and appears to have become well embedded in psychiatric nursing culture. *Well I think I'm quite non-judgemental. I do, I do read the files and we discuss people's behaviour, but I look at it as, as they've got personality disorder, and we're here to treat them. Not to judge them, and we have to work, work through this.*

Similar numbers of nurses argued that PD patients were 'sick', 'not well', have been 'diagnosed' and were suffering from a disorder that needs treatment. For one nurse it was the extremity and savagery of the index offences that confirmed that there was 'something wrong' with PD patients. Again, the outcome of this position was that nurses were able to justify to themselves the suppression of natural emotional reactions to what patients had done.

Kept tempers: not taking things personally

During the interviews quite a few staff talked about the need not to 'lose their cool', or 'personalize' the actions of patients. In fact 28 per cent of the nurses spoke about a need to contain or control their anger with patients, and 40 per cent spoke about feeling angry in various circumstances, many of which have been described more fully in the previous chapter. Some typically anger-arousing circumstances are discussed below.

Violence on the ward

The occurrence of a violent incident involving themselves or another nurse nearly always aroused angry feelings. This was the most frequent mention of nurses feeling angry, typically said by them to be a short-term, acute emotional response. These feelings were accentuated if the attack was planned in advance, if there was a pre-existing good, positive, therapeutically functioning relationship between patient and victim, and if the patient showed no remorse afterwards.

Verbal pressure

This involved being threatened, verbally abused or manipulated by patients, especially those patients with whom the nurses believed they had a good relationship. Constant demands from patients were found irritating and wearisome, particularly when coupled with either overt or covert threats to harm themselves. Being the target of unfounded, unjustified or trivial complaints by patients also angered nurses.

Index offences

In response to the index offence, typically when reading case notes, nurse anger would be accentuated if the index offence had been serious violence against vulnerable victims, had been planned in advance, treatment in hospital had been refused, no remorse had been shown, and pleasure had been taken in talking about it or blaming the victim.

These factors are clearly parallel to, if not the same as, those that prompt nurses to think about patients as evil monsters. The nurses did talk about becoming angry in other circumstances, typically around dealings with patients' relatives, or with the 'system', and these issues are explored else-where.

No nurses spoke of losing their temper within the context of a violent incident, and although nurses could react intensely to reading the case notes on a patient's index offence, the most acute form this took was that the patient would be ignored, or that a nurse would leave his or her job. Nurses did identify that loss of temper could easily take place when experiencing verbal abuse from patients, and as a typical expression the nurse would shout and swear at the patient in return. Becoming upset and angry in these circumstances is referred to by nurses as 'losing it'; 'losing your cool or your temper'; 'taking it personally'; 'responding positively'; 'internalising it'. This does happen on occasion: *Like if a patient starts shouting at you and you start shouting back, they'll shout higher, but if you just talk or try and calm them down, that can help them. You see some staff who just bawl and shout.* These events could be the culmination of a long period of relationship difficulty between patient and nurse because of borderline violence, continuous daily verbal criticism and abuse. Staff could become sensitized and touchy, having their 'back up' whenever the problematic patient came near. They describe being 'driven to distraction' and becoming completely unable to interact with the patient. General tiredness and stress can also make an emotional crisis more likely, and the content of the verbal abuse and criticism can be important in contributing to this. Patients can focus on a member of staff's weaknesses, tender spots, and sensitivities. Just as we all do when in a temper and arguing with someone – it's what makes marital arguments so foul – the weaknesses are known (and used). *And they tend to personally attack you to try and offend you, hurt you, work you up, try to make you do something.* Any available deficit of character or appearance can be highlighted and played upon by patients. Therefore a nurse who has low self-esteem and a poor level of self-confidence in certain areas is more likely to take offence and emotionally respond to abuse from a patient, particularly if this is targeted at their areas of weakness.

Talk that relates to the index offence is highly charged for nurses, and anything that patients say to indicate that they are not consciously remorseful is emotionally objectionable, for example criticizing other patients for what they have done themselves, or taking a major personal stand, getting on their high horse and taking offence at some trivial issue in which they think they have been hurt. *But yeah, there are some days where, say for example, they're complaining about something, really to you it's trivial, to them it's probably not, and or they've been having a go all day, and you just think, sometimes you just think, oh God I thought after what you've done.* Suppressed feelings about the patient's index offence can emerge on these occasions in a sudden loss of temper or angry outburst directed at the patient.

Some of the interviewed staff asserted over and over again that it was essential not to do this, regardless of the apparent provocation. Instead they recommended staying calm and reasoning with the patient, giving explanations for why things had happened or why they cannot have what they are demanding. One nurse describes how he did this on one tense occasion: *The other day we searched a patient's room, he'd got more possessions in his room than the hospital policy allowed. The staff told him about it, he got very angry, threatening, threatening violence, threatening to complain to the mental health act commissioners. I brought him in the office, sat him down, got the policy out, said look, the staff are doing what I tell them to do, I'm telling them to do it because this is what I've got to do because of the hospital policy, we've got no choice in the matter, you know, and this is what has to happen. And he went away and accepted it in the end.* There seems to be an underlying principle here of not downgrading, judging, dismissing, condemning, or destructively criticizing the PD patients. They are often hypersensitive and can be paranoid in their attitude, so as one nurse says: *Say the patient is demanding and demanding again and you say to him 'stop acting like a little boy'. You have lost a lot there. It will be construed, whether it's meant to be or not, it will be. Because these people, the majority of these people they talk to themselves, in their room.* Hostility from the patient is triggered so easily, and readily poisons the attempt to develop a nurse–patient relationship. In order to prevent this from happening, nurses strive to avoid confrontation in the first place by: treating patients with respect; explaining the rules; talking down in advance when someone is seen to be agitated; being pleasant and polite; being diplomatic; and being tactful. *Sometimes what you say to them can be taken the wrong way, and you have to be careful in that respect as well, you have to really think through what you're going to say to them, it's not going to offend them or make them angry in any way. And it's quite a bit of difference between somebody with a personality disorder and somebody like either you or me, in how you speak to them and how you can approach them. Body language as well if they'll interpret it things you know, that aren't really there, but, they'll pick up on it and they'll, they'll question you basically about things.*

Some nurses recommended the use of honest, objective, non-emotional feedback to patients about the effects of their behaviour. In doing so they manage to turn conflict into a therapeutic encounter, a learning opportunity for the patient concerned. *If someone's, you know, being verbally abusive to me for an hour, and then they get out of my hair for five minutes and come back and want something from me, then I just turn round and say, hang on a minute, you know, if I wasn't a nurse and you wasn't a patient then how would this work? I've got obligations you know through my professional conduct and I have to provide, but let's look at it realistically, you know outside you'd be told to get lost. You know and you kind of turn it round like that.* One nurse argued that it was essential to be honest and open with PD patients about the emotional effect they were having, and went on to say that this was important not just for managing the situation and one's own feelings, but also to provide a role model on how to manage productively and express angry feelings without an emotive argument.

Team support and individual clinical supervision are both seen by nurses as highly important in helping them to manage their own emotional reactions.

Partly this is about being able to ventilate those feelings so that the pressure reduces and they are more easily controlled during nurse–patient interaction. *But through support, supervision, female support group, talking to colleagues, supportive clinical team, it becomes a positive rather than a negative.* However if unresolved feelings about the patients' index offences are present, clinical supervision provides an arena within which nurses can ask themselves what they really feel, share it with others and work their way through it to a different emotional stance: *Part of training to be a nurse, it teaches you not to be judgemental and to be yourself and not put up a façade. And I'd like to think that I'm always of the same attitude and temperament and I have a professional outlook.* However there is also a lot the nurse team can practically do for each other – providing cover, sharing the burden, thereby protecting each other from emotional ignition: *Even, even knowing when to say, hold on I can't deal with that patient now, 'cos if I deal with him now, I'm going to fall out with him, I'm not going to be dealing with him appropriately, and just saying look, he's just asked me to do such and such can you do it, to another member of staff, and them doing it. I mean it's all those kinds of things sort of like, it's, I think it's about, you know, keeping yourself right. 'Cos it's so easy, you could so easily just lose your temper and just go in there and say* [lowers voice] *'just fuck off' kind of thing. And just blow all that professionalism and all that, you know, thing that you've built up over, over time.*

The nurses also talked about striving to keep things in perspective, seeing the big picture rather than getting overwhelmed by the moment. This meant taking a 'long-term perspective' on patient behaviour, seeing beyond what is happening in the here-and-now: *You experience a whole range of emotions. From fear, anger, distaste – but you have to keep in perspective that you're here to work and try to aid these people, at the end of the day.* In this sense the 'big picture' is the patients' treatment in hospital, the therapeutic work directed towards helping them overcome their problems, and the prevention of re-offending. As the phrase 'don't take it personally' hints, seeing the big picture can mean understanding that a patient's anger belongs to the nurse's position within the power structure of forensic psychiatric services and the role he or she plays, not to the nurse's attributes as a person. This understanding can enable nurses to keep their emotions in neutral while dealing with the situation objectively.

Psychological explanations of the behaviour of patients also help the nurses not to 'take it personally'. In this connection nurses did mention that the verbal abuse and anger of patients might be: anger displaced from elsewhere; a method learned from childhood of getting a desired state of affairs; a way of testing out nurses' commitments to them; or a means of provoking an emotional response.

Nurses with a positive overall attitude to PD were statistically more likely to have insight into their own emotional reactions and express awareness of ways to contain themselves (stay calm and reason with the patient, give honest feedback, turn conflict into therapy, utilize team support, see the big picture, psychologically understand the behaviour).

Avoiding disappointment and disenchantment

Some nurses report an emotional experience in their relationships with PD patients that can best be summed up as feelings of acute disappointment. The types of situation that give rise to these feelings are similar to those that provoke angry emotional responses from nurses. Feeling disappointed, like feeling angry, is also sometimes referred to by nurses as 'taking it personally'. Nurses' discourse on this topic also overlaps with their talk about building up trust with patients, and the difficulties in doing so.

Nurses make an emotional investment in their patients; they 'care for them' – not just neutral professional care, not a false façade, but a real commitment to other people via their work. That is their value system, and is usually why they entered nursing in the first place – in order to do meaningful, and morally valuable work. Because of this, nurses make a really hard effort to develop relationships with patients that express that caring ethic. This is not quite the same issue as trusting patients to clean their room, etc. Although contracts and promises can be made here too, and be broken leaving nurses feeling disappointed. These are overt formal promises that anyone can be expected to break from time to time. The relationship contract, which is covert, unspecified and more emotive, may merge into this but is essentially quite different and far more personal.

It is this commitment that PD patients trample on, leaving nurses feeling let down, betrayed, conned, etc. *To think that you put a lot of work in to try and get through to them and it wasn't appreciated and it wasn't, some of it was in vain, you know.* Something precious has been offered and given, something that nurses cannot ever, really, be paid to do. Something in addition to what they are remunerated for, which is not in their terms and conditions of employment. If the patients appeared to have accepted it and entered the contract of a genuine, caring, therapeutic relationship, the nurses believed in it and acted according to it – that is, until there was a crisis and the patients displayed behaviour that made nurses think they had only been acting all along. *You can be working with somebody for months and probably years and you might think you're getting somewhere and something happens and you get a big set back. And that can be difficult to, to deal with.* This nurse then talked about his feelings of betrayal when a patient, with whom he thought he had a good relationship, threatened him: *From my experience it's quite often patients you're perhaps close to . . . and for whatever reason they lose their temper, or sort of turn . . . it's almost like, well it is in a way a break down of that relationship, when it's you that they turn on.* This nurse's use of the word 'close' demonstrates the feelings of intimate knowledge and mutual trust that are part of a good nurse–patient relationship. When that relationship is challenged and effectively spurned by the patient, the nurse is left feeling shocked and disappointed. *You think that, I mean some-times you can think that you're getting somewhere and you really are building a relationship, and . . . you discover their manipulation and you think oh, God, you know, it's all been like a lie, the whole thing's a lie kind of thing.*

Not every 'let down' experience is quite as emotionally powerful as this. It seems to depend upon the depth and duration of the pre-existing relationship with the patient concerned. 'Let down' experiences may even be vicarious – witnessing them happening to one's colleagues, or even just hearing about them, may be enough to evoke an attenuated version of the same disappoint-ment: *There's been a couple of cases where people have like, retired early or left the service because of attacks from patients. Quite often, I would imagine, they were patients who those people were, in the long run, trying to help, you know. I think that's the difficult thing to swallow sometimes as well.* The nurses' emotional investment is not just in the relationship itself, but also in the therapeutic process. They are highly committed to helping the patients to overcome their problems and improve their lives. So, when there are set-backs, or the patients sabotage their treatment, strong feelings of disappoint-ment may be experienced, with nurses saying that in their 'heart of hearts' they felt let down, and had to struggle to put their disappointment behind them. Examples that were given included patients who had made great therapeutic progress, overcoming a repetitive cycle of being so disturbed as to require seclusion, or being very close to transfer to a less secure environ-ment, but who 'pressed the self-destruct button', resulting in acute dis-appointment for the nurses who had worked hard with them.

The most productive technique used by nurses to manage these disappoint-ments was a combination of trying to understand the PD patient's behaviour, and persevering with building and rebuilding relationships. The 'let down' experience was understood in various ways. Some staff saw it as the displace-ment of the patient's anger from elsewhere, that it was because the nurse was in a close relationship with the patient that he bore the brunt of everything that went wrong for the patient. Therefore the staff task was to accept that this was part of the therapeutic process. Other staff saw these setbacks as a psychological defence mechanism, employed unconsciously by patients who could not cope with the anxieties raised by intimacy. They noted that such disappointments were particularly prone to occur just on the verge of success, or just as the relationship was becoming close, and that this had to be accepted by staff even if they felt it was 'a kick in the teeth'. Yet other staff saw this as a repetitive, life-long pattern that resulted from the patients' experience of being repeatedly abandoned by others. As such, the appropriate task for staff, regardless of how many times they were 'knocked down', was to come back the next day and, by doing so, assure the patients that someone was 'there for them'.

The nurse who said this then argued that staff just have to put any dis-appointment behind them and 'get on with it', starting again from the begin-ning to build up a relationship with the patients. This recommendation is echoed by others, who also argue that nurses need to constantly hold in mind the expectation that they will be let down. The benefit of this strategy seems to be that the shock and unpleasant surprise are taken out of any eventual disappointment. Crucially one nurse recommended that probable future disappointments needed to be 'learned about' (consciously known and predicted), 'adjusted to' (emotionally accepted without anger), and 'worked with' (used therapeutically in objective feedback and discussion with the patients).

Turning criticisms into advantages

Despite the painful nature of accepting criticism and complaints, many nurses were able to describe the benefits of encouraging patients to voice them. Nurses who assented to the proposition that part of their role was to encourage patients to express criticisms and complaints, were more likely to have a positive overall attitude to PD, demonstrating that accepting criticism in this way was one means by which nurses attained and maintained that attitude. The perceived benefits of encouraging criticisms and complaints were: ventilation, discovery, partnership, service improvement, therapy, justice, and increased patient self-esteem. Those nurses with a negative attitude tended only to perceive the downside of criticisms and complaints by patients, and expressed feelings of betrayal, victimization and anger.

Some nurses saw it as important that patients should 'get it off their chest' if they had a complaint, rather than brood about it and allow it to simmer underneath an apparently good relationship. A variety of reasons were given for this being 'a good thing'. Firstly, emotional expression was seen as good in its own right. There appeared to be a crude underlying psychological theory that all emotional expression is *genuine* because it is instinctive, uncontrolled, and therefore unshaped; and *good* on the grounds that nonexpression leads to a build up of emotional pressure that is then expressed in a more unproductive fashion elsewhere. A typical example given by the nurses were the patients' anger being expressed in physical violence or verbal abuse towards others: *The benefits of that approach is that we know where we stand with them and they let off steam and they don't build up pressure if you like, and any situation is resolved by speech rather than physically.* Facilitating the ventilation of complaints was therefore seen as a means by which the ward is kept calm. In addition, the voicing of a complaint and criticism gave staff the opportunity to inform patients of the reasons why the ward operated as it did (typically, security rules), thus legitimizing the rules in the eyes of the patients while at the same time treating the patients with respect. Again this was seen as promoting a calm, orderly environment.

Via the content of the criticism, nurses learned how the patient thought, not an easy matter as PD patients did not readily trust or confide in anyone. So the expression of what was on their minds, even if critical and hostile, assisted nurses in establishing more open relationships with them. Moreover, when the content of the complaint was known, it could be dealt with through a resolution of the difficulty or by explaining why things could not be changed. This in turn created a sense of partnership between nurses and patients as they dealt with the issues together. Being ready to listen to criticism and complaints strengthened that relationship, and fostered rapport, trust, honesty and mutual respect. Other nurses argued that, once the complaints of patients were known they could be tackled together, and that this could lead to positive improvements in the way care was delivered. Complaints also meant that inappropriate staff could be removed, as one nurse described: *I had a colleague who was sacked for professional misconduct, for striking a patient. The complaint was upheld and he lost his ticket, and I think they have done nursing a favour. I think that is positive that some one had the guts to do something about it.*

The process of getting criticisms and complaints into the open, then dealing with them, was therapeutic for patients and could be used by nurses to help patients make therapeutic progress. They learn appropriate emotional expression and self-regulation, how to exercise coping skills, be assertive and express themselves appropriately. Nurses described aiding and advising during this process. Some nurses also suggested that the opportunity to criticize empowered patients, encouraged them to think as individuals and become more confident that their views were listened to and respected. Lastly, for some of the staff the acceptance of criticisms and complaints was seen as a moral good in its own right, quite separately from what was accomplished by it. These nurses saw an objective and fair complaints procedure as a patients' right that was theirs as a matter of principle.

The association with positive attitude implies that seeing and welcoming complaints in this way – as ventilation, discovery, partnership, service improvement, therapy, justice, and increased patient self-esteem – contributes to accomplishing daily work in a manner that is positive for staff.

Beliefs about the cause and treatment of PD

Staff were specifically asked what they considered to be the cause of PD, and their responses to this question fell into four categories. The largest number of nurses asserted that PD had originated in some way from childhood experiences. A number of different overlapping themes emerged under this heading but could not be sufficiently separated for them to be individually quantified. Childhood and upbringing were the topics most frequently mentioned, and this further broke down into descriptions of 'bad things done to', 'good things lacking' and 'environment'. Although child abuse is mentioned as a causative factor, it is not the only factor nurses pointed to as responsible for the later development of a PD.

At the opposite pole was a small group of nurses who expressed a confident belief that PD had a 'nature' cause of one type or another. People talked in terms of 'in the genes', 'genetic', 'born like that', 'just the way they are', 'in their make up', etc. In the middle were a substantial number who either tended to feel that nature/nurture played fairly equal parts, or that nature was there but that nurture predominated. Thus, for example, you could genetically inherit an in-built predisposition to PD which could lie dormant or be not too disruptive to one's life if nurture was good. A traumatic childhood or dysfunctional family, on the other hand, would bring out a predisposition and together cause problems leading to that person being in hospital. For most people 'a mix of both' could affect one individual, but a very small number saw it more in terms of either/or, i.e. some might be born with it, some might acquire it through nurture.

There was an additional group of nurses with a diverse set of responses to this question, who could only be categorized as 'other'. They could name and talk about different theories, but were themselves uncommitted to any. This group included those who simply stated they did not know, did not feel there was enough evidence upon which to base a judgement, hadn't given it enough thought, or asserted that PD was a mental illness without further explanation.

Holding a nurture theory on the aetiology of PD was associated with a positive overall attitude. Initially, it was believed that if nurture was the cause, there would be scope for effective therapy and personal growth towards normality. However this explanation had to be discounted because there was no association between belief in a nurture cause and belief in the treatability of PD patients, although belief in treatability was itself independently very strongly associated with positive overall attitude. Perhaps, then, it is that nurses who believed in a nurture cause were more likely to see PD patients as fellow human beings with motivations, needs and desires shaped by their past, as opposed to biological organisms with their behaviour determined in advance by some form of instinct.

All interviewees were asked whether they considered that PD patients were treatable. Responses to the question on treatability were coded into three categories: yes or mostly yes; some or to some degree; no or mostly no. As already mentioned, there was a very highly significant relationship between views on treatability and overall attitude, with positive nurses being more likely to believe in treatability. Despite this high correlation, there were substantial numbers of overall positive attitude nurses who had weak or no belief in treatability, and there were also substantial numbers of overall negative nurses who believed that some or most PD patients were treatable.

When views on treatability were compared with grade and hospital, similar patterns emerged to those displayed by overall attitude (Ashworth Hospital staff, and lower grades being more cynical about treatment efficacy). However there was no relationship to the gender of the nurse, whereas overall attitude was better among female nurses. This is indicative that belief in treatability is not the only driver of overall nurse attitude to PD. Examination of the responses by the current unit does show that PD unit nurses have a stronger level of belief in treatability. However, there are nurses who work on the PD units (14 per cent of those who work there) who definitively believe that most or all PD patients are untreatable.

If they affirmed that treatment could be effective in any way, nurses were asked what forms were appropriate for PD patients. Their responses were then roughly categorized. As this supplementary question was only asked of those who had some belief in treatability, it was not possible to relate the answers to overall attitude to PD patients. A number of nurses made generic replies to this question, simply specifying groups or individual work. Responses were not always well articulated, but it did appear that cognitive-behavioural therapy was well known and recommended by nurses. However, it was not always mentioned by name, and many of the replies categorized under this heading concerned teaching patients the effects of their behaviour on others, giving them feedback, or training them in methods of regulating their emotions. Although these were all counted as examples of cognitive-behavioural work, some might have been equally well categorized as therapeutic community methods. The latter were explicitly endorsed only by a small number of nurses, and even fewer nurses mentioned psychodynamic psychotherapy. It was surprising to find so many references to chemotherapy, as this is not a widely recognized treatment for PD. However, virtually all these were from unqualified nursing staff, who would have received little or no training in psychiatric treatment. Aspects of the organization and management of nursing care were themselves seen as therapeutic approaches – for example, a consistent nursing approach, ward structure, staff as role models. This topic is explored more thoroughly in a subsequent chapter.

A number of difficulties or hurdles in the delivery of effective treatment to PD patients were mentioned by nurses. These included: a lack of knowledge about what treatment works; the need for persistence in the face of difficulties and setbacks; difficulty in assessing the outcome of therapy in the hospital setting; apparent progress that could just be pretence in order to get discharged; and patients becoming institutionalized after a number of years in hospital. However, the most frequently mentioned difficulty was treatment refusal. Most often this was a declaration that some patients were not willing to engage in treatment at all and that, if this was the case, there was little that the hospital, or the nurses in it, could do. Nurses described how patients could avoid treatment in many different ways: simple refusal; presence in groups without real engagement; prioritizing other appointments and activities; agreeing to see one profession but not another; starting and then discontinuing treatments. This issue blended into questions about where PD patients should be cared for, with many nurses asserting that those who refuse treatment should be maintained within the prison system.

Under the present system, many pointed out that a patient could refuse treatment for years and years, and yet the hospital could not send them to prison. Other nurses saw resistance to treatment, particularly in new patients, as a hurdle that could be overcome, and talked about doing this by a gradual process of drawing patients into less threatening activities. It was acknowledged that this process could itself take years.

Some nurses, even those who had a strong belief in treatability, wondered how deep an impact any form of therapy could have on the PD patient. This was expressed in a number of thoughtful ways, for example 'you can alter behaviour but not personality', or 'patients can come to terms with it, but not be treated'. Running through these comments (and others like them) were reservations about the nature of the behavioural changes that are accomplished through therapy, that they are not as thoroughgoing or fundamental as nurses would really wish them to be, and that the disorder of personality cannot, in some very real sense, be undone.

Given the strong association between belief in treatability and positive attitude, it was important to try to establish how nurses had arrived at their positions. When asked what had shaped their opinion on treatability, the overwhelmingly dominant reply was experience – both for those who believed and those who did not. Many examples of successes and failures were given. Typical success stories were about patients who had shown positive changes on the ward over a period of time (e.g. 'Actually seeing them as they go out and you think well, he's a different chap to when he came in'), or who were discharged and did not return. Typical failure stories were of patients who had not changed over many years (e.g. 'he's been here for, God knows, 20 years or something, and if anything he's worse than when he first came in'), or who were discharged and subsequently readmitted. As might be expected, those nurses who believed in the treatability of PD patients provided more success stories. However, the question remains why nurses working at the same hospitals, caring for the same patients, came to such divergent opinions based on their experience? This seems to imply that belief in treatability perhaps impacts on the interpretations that nurses give to their experiences, or that positive nurses selectively attend to successes rather than failures while negative nurses do the reverse. Success and failure stories were further examined to see if cynical nurses saw treatment success more in terms of discharge than improvement on the ward, i.e. they had a more stringent criteria as to what counted as success. However, there was no relationship between these variables.

Several other factors were mentioned by nurses as shaping their views on treatability. As with experience, these factors could result in optimism or pessimism. Talk from other nurses was felt by some to have been an influence. This worked both ways, with some nurses declaring that what other nurses had said to them made them more cynical (e.g. 'just through things that staff have said, you know, that they can't be treated, that they are just the way they are'), whereas others reported the reverse (e.g. 'I've also been told by staff who have been working with patients for a very long time, the changes that have taken place, from let's say two years ago to now, with particular patients'). Courses and training formed another source of influence, but again this could cut both ways. Some nurses had clearly received a powerfully cynical message from their educators about the treatability of PD patients, whereas others had been enlivened and enthused by their experiences. Personal reading was also influential, but again the overall impact was ambivalent, with some nurses becoming more optimistic and others less so, depending on what they had read and accepted.

There were other sources of influence that appeared to have exerted a predominantly negative impact on belief in treatability. Being manipulated, let down, or attacked by PD patients was one of these. One nurse explained that the 'intense presence of PDs all the time' shaped his views towards absolute treatment pessimism, and concluded that 'there is very little a hospital like this can actually do for (them)'. Another described how experiences of being let down had led him to despair about the efficacy of treatment: *You've got that belief in your own head, then you give them so much help, you dig away and dig away, and they spit in your face. And you think what am I, what is the purpose?* It would appear from these comments and others that nurses' natural emotional reactions to the behaviour of PD patients colours their opinion about treatability, even though there is no logical connection. Of course, PD patients exhibit these difficult behaviours, but that is why they are considered to have a mental disorder and be in need of treatment. The other factor that caused nurses to doubt treatment efficacy was their perception of their inability to change themselves, with typical declarations being 'you just couldn't change me' or 'you are what you are', leading to the conclusion that the treatment of PD is futile.

A couple of items were mentioned by small numbers of nurses as positively influencing their beliefs in the treatability of PD patients. A working environment in which up-to-date research-based treatment methods are being applied to PD patients appeared to generate more optimistic attitudes. Other nurses mentioned that, for them, belief in treatability was a consequence of their personal ethical position, whether that was religious or philosophical. *I've always had a positive attitude towards human beings anyway. Yeah I've always felt that you know that if you can bring out the best in somebody, nobody is all bad, and there's the best, and you know if you can home in on that and use that.*

Diminished responsibility for actions

The nurses were asked if patients with personality disorder were responsible for their actions and were virtually unanimous that PD patients are responsible either completely or to some degree. A number of variant positions were identifiable, but the largest proportion clearly considered PD patients (or most PD patients) responsible, to a certain extent, for whatever they do. This view sharply contrasts with the location of the High Security Hospitals within the criminal justice system. Patients have largely been sent to those hospitals because they are considered to be mentally disordered and not responsible for their actions. Yet it is clear, once they arrive within the forensic psychiatric system, that they are considered by nearly all the nursing staff to be at the very least partly responsible for their actions. Some of the nurses reflected on the way these positions did not fit logically together. They couldn't square their desire to say that PD patients were responsible, with their commitment to treating them in hospital and considering them mentally disordered: *It's a hard one for me to answer. I think I've gone round the houses on it.* In order to make things clear some are reduced to statements which make no obvious sense: *At the moment of the incident, they might not have been in control through various things – drugs, alcohol, whatever – but they are responsible.*

Also notable is the fact that judgements of PD patients' responsibility bear no statistical relationship whatsoever to overall attitude to PD, whether that be positive or negative. This lack of relationship is maintained irrespective of how the 'responsibility judgements' are grouped. Given that it is clear that certain PD patients are condemned by some nurses who are angered by their index offences and behaviour on the ward, it might have been expected that the attribution of responsibility would be linked to a negative attitude. However, this was not the case, and nurses made their 'responsibility judgements' on the basis of a different and separate pattern of reasoned argument. It is some of these underlying arguments and rationales that *were* associated with overall attitude to PD.

A significant number of nurses argued that everybody was responsible for what they did, with many of them saying that they had always considered this to be the case as a matter of personal philosophy or fundamental belief. This viewpoint was so strongly held and expressed that a few nurses making this argument went as far as to argue that patients who were actively psychotic were still responsible for their index offences. There was no relationship between the expression of this viewpoint and overall attitude to PD, gender, grade or hospital. However, this judgement was related to age, it being held and expressed more often by younger nurses.

Other nurses argued that PD patients were responsible because they were cognitively competent. They expressed this body of reasoning in a number of different ways, and the use of this type of argument was very highly related to a negative overall attitude to PD. The most common way in which this argument was articulated was for the nurse to say 'they know what they are doing'. This point was made by many nurses, and their additional comments implied that the PD patients were not confused or muddled, and were fully aware of what they did and the fact that it was wrong. Others voiced this argument differently, saying that PD patients were not ill and, more specifically, were not deluded or hallucinated. Many nurses drew a clean and clear distinction here between offenders who suffered from psychotic illnesses and were not responsible, and those who were simply PD: *I feel that they're responsible 'cos it's not, unlike mental illness, a personality; people with mental illness actually do lose touch with reality. Personality disorder patients, I feel, don't lose touch with reality, they always, they have a goal in mind for a particular reason however small or large, to do it whether it be for their own self-indulgence or to gain, to gain whatever.* Yet other nurses who maintained the same overall position pointed to the fact that the behaviour of PD patients was goal-directed, planned and self-oriented: *Well they seem to think about what they're doing, they plan everything they're doing, so I'd say they are responsible, yes.* This view was confirmed for nurses when patients used their illness consciously as an excuse (e.g. ''Cos we've had patients say, I'm saying this because I'm a PD so I can say things like this. Well obviously he knows') or when patients rationally and consistently argued that they were not to blame, thus displaying an awareness of what they had done (e.g. 'Because they have reasons, they seem to have reasons for why they actually did that, and although they might be blaming somebody else, the fact that they are able to stick to a reason means they are responsible. They are conscious of the act').

Some nurses voiced a number of arguments that could be considered as portraying a view of the PD patient as having incomplete or eroded cognitive competence. Nurses who made this type of argument were not in general suggesting that PD patients had no responsibility at all, but that their responsibility was slightly diminished. This position was not generally associated with a positive attitude to PD, as might have been expected, given the link between a cognitive competence viewpoint and negative attitude. However, there was one important exception to this, which will be described below.

Three ways in which nurses reasoned that PD patients had diminished responsibility had no association with attitude. Some nurses argued that where there was a co-existing mental illness, specifically a psychosis, then PD patients could not be considered responsible for their actions. For 8 of the 10 nurses using this argument, this was seen as the only conceivable excusing factor, with the remaining PD patients being seen as fully responsible without exception. Other nurses considered PD itself to be an illness that excused behaviour (e.g. 'They are not well because they're mentally disturbed. How do you control your behaviour if you're mentally disturbed? They probably don't know what they're doing'). Three nurses mentioned a genetic cause for PD when making this argument. Yet others suggested that an impulsive action or index offence should be seen as less culpable: *But I think that, if they were having a flash back, or even in moments of extreme anger, sometimes I think they do lose the ability, or some of them can lose the ability, to control what they're doing, or to realize what they're doing.*

However, there was a small group of staff that argued in a distinctive way for the diminished responsibility of PD patients, suggesting that they had an incomplete or warped perspective on the world, significantly different from that of ordinary people. This was voiced in a variety of ways, with one person arguing, for example, that patients may know what they are doing, but that their view is not fully informed, they don't understand or have an overview of their own behaviour, its patterns and origins. Therefore although they are responsible they are not fully responsible. Others pointed to the abusive childhoods some PD patients had endured, described them in shocking detail and asked 'how responsible can he be?', or reflected that this 'is the only behaviour they know', or that the choices the patients had were not like those of 'you and I'. Yet others stated explicitly that PD patients had an altered perception of the world, 'a different slant or view on what is normal within society', and that this excused their behaviour, because they 'haven't got the insight' or 'don't realize what they are actually doing'. Later in the interview the same nurse suggested that 'they don't think the same way as perhaps I do about things' and that social circumstances, events, and their environment all affect PD patients differently than they do other people. These statements perhaps reflect the fact that the social world is a strange place when viewed from the PD patient's standpoint. The use of these arguments was highly correlated with an overall positive attitude to PD.

Parental identification

Completely unexpectedly, many of the staff interviewed spoke about being like parents towards PD patients. The following extended quotation from one of the interviews is a good example: *I think that the majority of the PDs that I work with, certainly here, is that identity is an issue. Trying to find out who they are, what they are and finding positive role models within the staffing. Also to trust staff is very very important to them. So the usual boundaries around, you know, demonstrating a positive adultness about them, is really important. That's not always what I see around me but that's what they require. They require sort of positive, i.e. parenting in the staffing and that's, that's sometimes very very difficult for staff to do because of pressures and because of the system and what have you. But that's what they're searching for, so therefore it doesn't always happen, so as a result you tend to get lots of problems with PDs.*

The way in which nurses felt that they took a parental role towards PD patients broke into four components: love, trust, authority, and role model. In terms of 'love', nurses felt that they provided parental care, understanding and nurturance, with many linking this to the absence of such care and attention during the patient's childhood. When stating this they use words and phrases like 'mothering', 'nurturing' or 'want to sort of just take them back to their childhood and just change everything for them'. Others linked this to identification issues. They saw the PD patient as 'like' their son or daughter in certain respects, saying, for example, that *having children of my own has helped me with these type of patients, in bringing up three sons that they had their moods, their swings, and, I relate a lot of their*

ways to the ways of children and teenagers. The PD patients exhibited behaviours that reminded them of their children, or caused them to consider
that their child might encounter similar difficulties. In a sense they were
realizing how close we all are as human beings to the PD experience, and
how narrowly we are separated from it.

For some of the nurses, taking the parental role, whether they expressed
this as being motherly or fatherly, meant that patients would trust them,
have confidence in them, and confide in them. Again, this was sometimes
seen in terms of providing something for patients which had been lacking
during their childhood, when *All the people they're supposed to trust, their
parents, their families, people that, you know, run homes, children's homes
and things like that, they haven't been able to trust them bastards, they screwed
round with their brains, their bodies and their, all their . . . you know.*

In terms of authority, nurses talked about the parental role in setting
limits, laying down boundaries, applying rules for behaviour, and being a
source for the determination of right and wrong. Within this context
nurses spoke of the respect that patients were then willing to give in this
type of relationship. Nurses also connected being parental to the provision
of a role model for patients to follow and copy. Again, just as with love
and trust, nurses linked this to the things that had been missing in the PD
patients' childhoods, where those in the real parental role had been unstable,
chaotic, changeable and volatile.

There was a very strong relationship between expressions of parental
attitudes and positive attitudes to PD overall. It may be that the experience
of having adolescent children encourages nurses to think in this way, but
there was no relationship between these expressions and the age of the
nurse. However there is a strong link to gender, with female nurses being
much more likely to express this role relationship. Thus, for nurses, identifying themselves as a parent towards PD patients seems to be one possible way
in which nurses maintained a positive overall attitude. There were other
identifications that were clearly not so productive, and in the previous
chapter we saw that identifying oneself or one's child with the victim of
the index offence was likely to arouse feelings of anger and fear, and make
it difficult to interact with PD patients.

Seeing themselves in the parent role was not the same for nurses as seeing
PD patients as similar to children. There were some nurses who expressed
this view, drawing out the similarity in two ways. Some saw the PD patients
as lovable little rogues, conveying a kind, warm appreciation of the patient,
coupled with an understanding and sympathetic attitude to their behaviour,
using words like 'naughty' and 'mischief'. Others saw them as nasty little
brats, and these references were less warm and carried derogatory connota-
tions. Using adjectives such as 'spoilt', 'greedy', 'childish', 'dummy coming
out of the pram', 'tantrums', and 'selfishness', the nurses' statements convey
a feeling of resentment, anger and rejection. There were, however, insufficient

numbers of cases of these two forms of child analogy to assess separately their individual relationship to overall attitude. Together, there was no association with attitude to PD.

Summary

The difficulties facing staff who care for and treat PD patients are enormous, and constitute a significant personal challenge for the psychiatric professional of any discipline. Those staff who manage the challenge positively, enjoy their work, feel safe and secure, are accepting towards patients, have a sense of purpose and are enthusiastic, have particular ways of dealing with work-related issues. Some of these ways have been discovered and detailed by this research, but they are not wholly separable – some being interdependent and others synergistic. They consist of beliefs, moral commitments, skilled interpersonal actions, cognitive self-management strategies, specific applied knowledge, and skilled teamwork. They are, in the order in which this chapter has introduced them:

Professionalism   A commitment to the idea that professionals provide a high standard service regardless of who the client is or what has been done. For many in this study this was, specifically, an allegiance to nursing professionalism, allowing them to focus on the care and treatment of patients.

Individualized care   An allegiance to the idea that everyone is unique and has to be understood as the product of his or her own personal history, coupled with a rejection of grouping, labelling, herding and stereotyping.

Prevention   A primary commitment to the prevention of further crime and harm to others, to look forward rather than backward.

Illness   Seeing patients' behaviour as symptomatic of an illness, thereby absolving them from blame.

Abuse reminder   Actively remembering and calling to mind the patient's history of abuse and suffering, to set against past or current actions.

Universal humanity   Recalling that we, including PD patients, are members of the human race and are deserving of equality, human rights, compassion and pity.

Behaviour/person split   Drawing a distinction between PD patients' behaviour, which could be seen as bad, and the patients themselves, who are not.

Person-now   Concentrating and focusing attention on persons as they are now, their current behaviour and relationship with them.

Person-first   Meeting the patients first, getting to know them as persons, before finding out about their index offences or reading the case notes. Thus balancing the reality of the patients as individual human beings against the knowledge of what they have done.

Non-judgementalism   Adherence to an ethic that stresses a refusal to judge any patient for anything. Also a strategy thought to result in therapeutic change in patients.

Reasoning   Staying calm and reasoning with the disturbed patients, explaining the reasons behind restrictions, etc. If possible, doing this in a respectful way before the patients become angry and agitated, thus avoiding confrontation.

Feedback   Giving objective, unemotional feedback to patients about the effects of their behaviour.

Reciprocal emotional pumping   Taking the bad feelings engendered by the patients and their behaviour, and expressing them to colleagues rather than to the patients. Similarly, taking supportive feelings from colleagues and converting them into personal strength in the encounter with the patients.

Timeshare   Sharing the burden of interacting with a difficult patient between the nursing team.

Big picture   Seeing beyond what is happening in the here-and-now, taking a 'long-term perspective' on patient behaviour.

Understand   Striving for psychological understanding and interpretation of PD patients' behaviour, using a range of models and explanations. Accepting that their perspective of the world is warped and different – a cognitive incompetence model.

Expectation   Anticipating that PD patients are likely to disappoint and let down their carers.

Perseverance   Willingness to try again after failure, repeatedly, dogged determination, patience.

Facilitating complaints   For ventilation, discovery, nurse–patient partnership, service improvement, justice, and therapy.

Nurture cause   Belief in a nurture cause of PD.

Treatment efficacy   Belief in treatment efficacy.

Parent identification   Viewing oneself as in a parental role towards patients (love, trust, authority, role model).

The description of these methods in a systematic way for the first time means that there is scope to train staff in their use, thus promoting a long-term positive approach to the care and management of PD patients. They do not, however, exist in a vacuum. The organizational context can either support or hinder their use. How the nursing team works together, how it relates to the hospital management and other psychiatric professions, etc., are all areas where positive attitudes can be promoted or undermined. We turn to these issues in the next chapter.

5 A supportive organization and team

Positive attitudes to PD patients cannot solely be conceived as the isolated production of an individual member of staff. As the previous chapter showed, individual staff may use different techniques to adjust to the work with PD patients. However, that is not the whole story, as the questionnaire survey demonstrated in showing that staff attitudes were 30 per cent influenced by the hospital within which they worked. Obviously hospital culture itself must therefore be exerting some form of influence. The interviews of staff contained sufficient detail to permit an elaboration of those influences and how they work, and this chapter will describe mechanisms which divide roughly into two broad areas: how the whole staff of the hospital, as a social group, manages conflict; and how the organization prepares and supports individuals for work with PD patients.

One form in which the pathology of PD patients is expressed is that of manipulative behaviour, and one subtype of that behaviour is 'dividing' – the creation of antagonism and conflict between others by the telling of lies, falsehoods or exaggerations of different sorts to different parties. This tendency to divide may be wielded consciously or unconsciously by the PD patient, and feeds upon any pre-existing splits and divisions within social groups that can most readily be widened and extended. The consequences for the organization of the hospital are profound, as divisions naturally exist between grades of nurses, between nurses and their managers, and between the different psychiatric professions working as part of the multi-disciplinary care team. Thus the pathology of PD patients finds expression in the social relations between these subgroups – a process that can be either hindered or facilitated by the ways in which the organization works (or doesn't work) as a whole.

The other way in which the organization impacts upon attitudes to PD is through how it prepares staff to work with PD patients, and then supports them once they are engaged in that work. Here the two critical areas are training (basic professional education, induction to the hospital, and specialist PD-related courses), and clinical supervision. Both areas require the investment of resources, and considerable organizational talent to implement them within the context of a busy hospital. Yet the consequences of failure to do so can have a dramatic impact on the attitudes of staff, and the level of care that patients receive.

Violence and nursing team cohesion

Paradoxically, one form of behaviour of PD patients that nurses find difficult to manage also serves to draw together the nursing team on the ward. For nurses, the thing that makes it feasible to work within such a threatening environment is the knowledge that the rest of the nursing team will provide support and backup if an incident occurs. Each hospital has a sophisticated system that means that large numbers of staff will arrive very quickly once the alarm bells have been rung. *You get people everywhere coming from everywhere, and that gives you a feeling of security, but the most thing that gave me a secure feeling that day, was working on this ward with my team that I was working with.* The external threat from patients thus creates high levels of team cohesion and trust, which are themselves strengthened each time support is given or received. To rush to give help and support becomes the iron law of nursing life – indeed, a condition of team membership.

This factor may go some way towards explaining several common phenomena within the hospitals. Firstly, the separation and distance between nurses and their managers. On leaving the rank and file who are exposed to daily threat, those promoted to managers are no longer considered to be part of 'the team', but are potential sources of further threats to nurses' sense of control over the work environment and, hence, to their feelings of security. Secondly, the resistance of the nursing team to change from outside may also be a consequence of rigid and continuously rewarded cohesion to the 'team line'. Thirdly, nurses may find it difficult to criticize each other or to root out bad practice, insofar as it is perpetrated by those who, in other contexts, have come to the nurse's aid at high risk to themselves.

Nurses took great pride in the fact that they could often avoid violence by verbal means. Several slightly different approaches were mentioned, using the words 'talk down', 'diffusion', 'de-escalation', etc. These are techniques that are taught as parts of basic nurse training and of control and restraint courses.

- Identifying incipient violence and getting the patient to express the problem verbally, so that ventilation occurs and things can be explained or resolved.
- Using neutral discussion that is not prejudged; refraining from shouting or losing control; staying calm; not responding to abuse and criticism with anger; exploring the anger-causing issue from different perspectives.
- Using a prior, well-established good relationship with patients so that they can confide and talk, rather than become aggressive.
- Diverting the patient off the anger-causing topic onto another, more neutral and less emotional issue.

- Being polite and respectful to the patient as an individual, rather than dismissing or judging the patient's anger.
- Suggesting other ways of coping with the situation.

Utilizing these approaches under the imminent threat of physical violence cannot always be easy, but nurses stated that this was their preferred method of dealing with the problem, regarding it as a 'better skill' than the use of physical restraint. What is more, being able to successfully 'talk down' a patient who is angry was reported to be a highly rewarding (albeit stressful) experience, and interviewees were pleased to relate some of their successes: *And usually within 10 minutes you can have somebody who's near exploding, calm down, look at things from a different perspective, and be able to walk out and say thanks, actually thank you for, sort of like, allowing him to express in that way, you know.*

All nurses in the High Security Hospitals receive training in control and restraint techniques, and this is mentioned by many of them in relation to dealing with violence. It is clear that knowledge and training in these techniques adds to nurses' confidence and security in dealing with violent incidents. Others pointed out that a certain level of toughness is required of nurses who work in these environments. Nurses have to be able to stand their ground, manage a confrontation rather than avoid it, and show that they have not been intimidated following an incident of any kind. Some express this as not being afraid of the patients; others speak of repressing and hiding fear from the patients. *You've got to show that you're not affected by it. You've got to, you've got to show the personality disorder patient that you're not influenced by them. You've just got to stand firm and show that, you know, you're in control.* Several interviewees referred to nurses who had not been able to handle the level of stress provoked by the constant threat of violence, and had had to leave the High Security Hospitals because they 'sort of had a breakdown' or became 'nervous wrecks'. Because the nursing team is unsure how any new member of staff is going to be able to cope with serious violence, and because they are so dependent on each other for support, in some cases incorporation as a fully-fledged member of the nursing team is dependent on showing some toughness and ability to cope. Along these lines one nurse said: *You're not really accepted at all until you've been involved in your first incident. Until they've seen you run to the alarm bells like everybody else. Until they've seen you control and restrain a difficult patient.*

Whether violence was successfully de-escalated and avoided, or whether it had to be contained using physical restraint and seclusion, it is clear that it represented an external threat to the nursing team that was not shared with managers or other members of the multidisciplinary team. As a consequence of being dependent on each other for basic physical safety, in an environment populated by PD patients who had already demonstrated their capacity to commit serious crimes, the nursing team pulled together, becoming strongly cohesive and standing shoulder to shoulder.

Nursing assistants as ward team members

This cohesion was further demonstrated in that, although there was an obvious division in the ward-based nursing team between qualified and unqualified staff, patients were not able to readily exploit that division as they did between other groups. Generally speaking, nursing assistants (unqualified nurses, just over 40 per cent of the nursing staff) looked to the qualified nurses for information, guidance and advice. In response to some interview questions, they would commonly say they were not qualified to give an answer. Typically this was in response to questions about the cause of PD, treatment, medication, diagnosis, the organization of care, etc. When they did voice an opinion on such matters, they referred to having gained the knowledge through 'speaking to the qualified staff', 'asking questions' and taking 'advantage of their knowledge'. Qualified staff, therefore, picked up the responsibility for training nursing assistants, who referred to them as 'the most valuable source of information and training'. This includes not just instruction in theoretical knowledge, but also guidance on managing patients and feedback on any successful activity, such as de-escalating aggressive patients: *I actually brought him down on my own just by talking calmly to him. When you are face to face with somebody twice the size of you it can get quite worrying. You tend to be a little bit quiet afterwards and the qualified staff just took me to one side, calmed me down a bit. Basically I was just praised for how I handled the situation.*

There are tensions in the relationship between qualified and unqualified nursing staff, but in the face of the external threat from patients, these seem to recede into the background. For example, experienced nursing assistants could have a rather jaundiced view about staff who came to the High Security Hospitals shortly after qualifying. They considered that basic nurse education did not adequately prepare them to take charge of looking after PD patients, and commented that they had seen newly qualified nurses who 'seemed to think they were the next messiah' and could 'wave a magic wand' and cure anybody. With wry humour the same nursing assistant pointed out that the patients 'soon pick up on this' and have them 'jumping through hoops'. They were put in the difficult position (on occasion) of knowing better than those ostensibly in charge of them, creating a sense of awkwardness when they had to point things out. Relationships are not always smooth. Nursing assistants could be made aware of their lower status in a number of ways. For example, qualified staff could refuse to deal with them over the phone, asking for the nurse in charge, even for such trivia as the borrowing of a loaf of bread. Nevertheless, many responses (e.g. 'we're all a team so it shouldn't make a difference') show that team cohesion can be good, overcoming the rather artificial divisions introduced by status and hierarchy.

Throughout qualified nurses offered many glowing tributes to the work of nursing assistants. For example, 'there are some extremely able nursing assistants who can offer a lot in this environment' and 'I have worked with some damned fine nursing assistants'. These are only two of a very large number of similar statements.

Many qualified nurses commented that personal manner and approach in dealing with PD patients are more important than a qualification, referring to this as 'natural ability', and remarking that, in this area, some nursing assistants are 'better than the qualified' staff. Examination of the context of these remarks showed that the abilities in view were those of preventing daily trouble, and getting cooperation from patients in daily living activities. It made the working day easier to have staff whose manner did not produce conflict or confrontation and who could smooth the activities of the day.

However, contrary to the claim that these were 'natural abilities', the valued nursing assistant characteristics described by qualified staff were good interpersonal skills of the type taught in psychiatric nursing courses. These included: a good rapport with patients; an ability to winkle out of patients what is upsetting them; eliciting confidence and trust from patients; being diplomatic rather than sharp in manner; having better interaction or people skills. The truth is probably a mixture of both claims, some people being naturally more interpersonally skilful in this way, and others having acquired such skills through training and experience.

Although the value of these personal qualities was widely recognized by qualified nursing staff, they were also aware of the fact that they had more relevant experience in psychiatry to draw upon when dealing with PD patients. They also felt they had more knowledge, and knew better what to expect from PD patients, especially in contrast to newly hired unqualified staff whom they felt 'didn't have any idea'. Experienced nursing assistants were highly valued, but the inexperienced were not, being seen rather as a hindrance or even as a potential disaster (e.g. 'catalyst for catastrophe' was the view of one nurse). Several of the nurses interviewed referred to a series of events that had taken place involving a young, female, single parent nursing assistant who was inveigled into a 'conditioned' relationship by a PD patient. He started by giving her little gifts, firstly for herself, then for her children, and then tried to use this as leverage to create a personal relationship with her. Young nursing assistants were seen as particularly vulnerable in this way, and in need of careful supervision from, and protection by, the qualified staff. Several nurses recommend that all nursing assistants should be older, and certainly not school leavers. Two qualities were seen as more likely to occur among older unqualified staff: from experience of being conned and lied to, a certain wariness that comes with maturity; and a breadth of life experience, giving the person a wider conversational repertoire to utilize in interaction with patients.

In short, although some nursing assistants saw qualified staff as over-confident or overbearing, and some qualified staff saw some nursing assistants as inexperienced or vulnerable, the majority opinion was one of high mutual regard and common identity. The two groups expressed a willingness and capacity to learn from each other and support each other, and it seems likely that this strong cohesion was at least partly produced through the external threat posed by the PD patients.

Conflict with management

Given the large political profile of the High Security Hospitals, plus the inquiry culture, the dangerousness of the patients, and being at the centre of legal challenge and debate about mental health legislation and practice, to be part of the management of such an institution must be supremely difficult. A few nurses recognized the difficulties that their managers experienced, with one saying that the High Security Hospitals 'are management nightmares'.

There were many generic comments in the interviews about managers either being 'supportive' or 'unsupportive'. By themselves these statements did not provide an understanding of the actions that nurses considered to be 'support' from management. However, many respondents expressed at great length what they meant by 'unsupportive' managers. These comments boiled down to conflict in three areas: being undermined, the handling of official complaints, and the manipulation of patients. In many cases the degree of stress and high feelings around these areas completely divided the ward-based team of the nurses from their non ward-based managerial colleagues.

Although the comments made by nurses about their managers were predominantly negative, some were positive, and many examples were given of good management practice. Nor were all the criticisms aimed by staff at their managers necessarily justified. However, clear evidence was gained from the interviews that the ways in which PD patients behaved generated particular pressures on the relationship between nurses and their managers, and that responses to these pressures were patterned, predictable, and not easy to overcome.

The biggest complaint that nurses had about their managers was that they undermined the authority of ward-based staff over the patients. These events typically arose when nurses 'said no' to patient requests, only to find subsequently that they had been overruled by those further up the nursing hierarchy. This might be the ward manager, or a nurse in a middle management position, or even on occasion the top managers and executives of the hospital. Nurses found such experiences very disheartening, feeling 'trodden upon', 'angry', 'devalued', 'forgotten', 'demoralized', 'frustrated', 'insecure', 'helpless', and that their efforts in patient care had been 'wasted'. Nurses quoted these events explicitly as reasons why they had no faith or trust in their managers.

Because PD patients seek immediate gratification of their wishes, or because they are always trying to uphold a fragile sense of self worth, when one nurse refuses them something they will go to another, sometimes further up the hierarchy. Thus PD patient behaviour constantly provides occasions upon which nurses can feel undermined. When nurses have been undermined in this way, they will often be more reluctant to say 'no' to patients in future, and are likely to follow a policy of appeasement: *Sometimes when you should be not stricter but more upfront, you think, oh I am not going to say that, I am not going to say no you can't have that because it won't be worth the trouble because they will only go and see somebody else and they will give it to them anyway, so why should I put my neck on the chopping block?* Nurses do not only become reluctant to say 'no' because they are intimidated by the patient and may be overruled; they also fear being seen by their managers as having done something wrong. This fear, regardless of its reality, acts as a brake on their nursing management of patients and situations, leading to an erosion of the ward rules and structure. Where the person who is doing the overruling is the ward manager, very serious situations can develop over a period of time, and the safety of patients, staff, and the public may come under threat. One nurse described how this had happened on a ward where he had worked. A new ward manager had been appointed who did not back up his staff in confronting PD patients, and the ward became almost self-governed by the patients: security rules were disregarded (e.g. rules on the use of knives), staff began to fear the patients and 'it was totally out of control'. These situations are retrievable by appropriate nursing action, as the same respondent then described: *That situation has changed. A new clinical nurse, clinical leader took over there, and sort of basically backed up staff, pulled in the boundaries, was consistent in their approach. The same patients up there, you know, are much more manageable now.*

The newer regimes at the High Security Hospitals are more liberal, and a greater emphasis is laid upon patients' human rights. Much of this new emphasis has flowed from the public inquiries, especially the Blom-Cooper Inquiry into Ashworth Hospital, which uncovered the inhumane treatment of patients by nurses. However, a consequence of this change in regime is that some nurses feel undermined by the process of change, that their control over their work situation has been eroded, and that those who know nothing about the job ('administrators' and 'those from other walks of life coming in as senior managers') are dictating the way they, as nurses, should run their wards. Yet this point of view is not correct. The reforms that followed the Blom-Cooper Inquiry were brought in by experienced psychiatric nurses who were fully knowledgeable and qualified to do so. And managers do have a right, indeed a clear responsibility, to say how nursing should be practised on the wards for which they are responsible.

Similar issues arise when a particular incident in which nurses were overruled is considered. One nurse described how a patient on a female ward asked to have a 'nought' haircut (completely shaved head). The nurses on the ward said 'no', on the grounds that this was not feminine and would make the patient look like a thug. They felt that this type of haircut contradicted their efforts to help their patient look normal, and that it would highlight the scars from self-inflicted wounds on her face. In response, some of the patients wrote to a senior manager, who wrote back saying that the patient could have the haircut she wanted. It is possible to see both sides to this argument, the nurses wishing to see patients look attractive, and the patients wanting to have their own choice of hairstyle. In such a situation it is the manager's responsibility to take the final decision. Therefore, nurses must expect to be overruled on occasion, and come to terms with the reality that managers have decision-making responsibilities. Instead, some nurses' beliefs about managers are deeply suspicious: *And it is terrible when you're on your own as regards, you've got the patients under you who's having a go, and trying to find every little chink in the armour. And you've got the management above that will quite happily back them up.*

There are means by which managers and nurses can make this awkward reality easier to handle. Managers could be reluctant to overrule ward nurses, and express that reluctance even when they do, giving a full explanation as to why. Nurses could expect that they might be overruled, and perhaps express their decisions in a more tentative form, as temporary, or for the moment, or until things can be further discussed with managers and the clinical team, etc. However, the ideal situation is that any differences among the professionals and their managers should be resolved in private discussion. Some nurses were able to give positive accounts, demonstrating that it is possible for clinical teams and their managers to work together to agree rules for patient conduct, thus avoiding from the beginning any occasion in which nurses can feel undermined. One nurse described how this had taken place on their ward, with a series of meetings being held between nurses and their managers, everyone being allowed to have their say, and clear guidelines for patient conduct defined and written down. Those guidelines were then explained to all the patients both as a group and individually.

Part of the problem for staff in this area is a lack of clarity about who is responsible for taking what type of decision. There are many decisions that front line staff can and should take, and there are others that should be referred to managers, or to particular officers of the institution (e.g. security matters). When it is not clear where spheres of responsibility lie, managers may seek to take all decisions so that they feel more in control, or wards and multidisciplinary teams can seek to become semi-independent, as happened notoriously on one ward at Ashworth Hospital (Fallon *et al.* 1999). One interviewee commented on the confusion over decision-making roles: *Unfortunately within a special hospital you can't make rules 'cos you get overruled by management, who tend to overrule all their own rules anyway.*

The dynamics of this whole process of 'undermining' are of great interest for the light they shed upon nurse–patient relationships, and because, in a sense, the nurse–patient relationship is being mirrored in the manager–nurse relationship. PD patients find being told 'no' a difficult experience, one to which they respond with catastrophic feelings of low self-esteem, worth, value, and loss of face (the thought that others perceive them as less worthy). The nurses respond in a similar fashion when being told 'no' by their managers, and a similarly catastrophic reaction can materialize. That this happens is neither mysterious nor surprising. For many PD patients self-esteem is a primary issue in all their interactions with nurses, a bias possibly acquired through a history of being abused and being made to feel thoroughly worthless. The prominence of the issue probably rubs off on the nurses, who become sensitized to any slight or implicit criticism from their managers. In addition, nurses are further sensitized by the volume and frequency of the verbal and physical abuse they receive from patients. No wonder their reaction to being contradicted by managers is so emotionally intense.

The official complaints system is another area where the behaviour of patients generates conflict between nurses and their managers. The complaints system, and patients' manipulation of it, have been analysed in a previous chapter. There it is described how patients used complaints based on unfounded allegations in order to have nursing staff, whom they consider undesirable, moved to other wards or suspended. Alternatively, they used the threat of making a complaint to intimidate nurses in order to gain something they desired. The complaints that were made can be on unbelievably trivial and petty issues, and the complaints investigation process caused nurses high levels of stress. On a more positive note, nurses perceived complaints to be: a basic human right; an opportunity for patients to express their feelings and grievances; a way for them to learn conflict resolution skills; a mechanism to prevent bullying between patients; and a means to improve the hospital service. Nurses expressed a strong preference for dealing with complaints informally at ward level, and many suggested one-to-one nurse conversations, or the ward community meetings, as the appropriate place for criticisms to be raised. Some nurses argued that unless complaints were positively encouraged at this stage, a greater number of formal complaints would result.

Those comments in the interviews that addressed the manager's role in the complaints process were largely critical. The criticisms were two-fold: firstly, that managers reacted too strongly (by means of suspensions and moves) to trivial complaints; and, secondly, that they expressed no concern and gave no support to nurses who were the targets, who might have felt upset, angry, guilty without due cause, and who were stressed and traumatized. It was described how one nurse had asked a patient to turn the television down, and that the patient then made an official complaint, arguing that he felt threatened by the nurse and wanted him moved off the ward. The nurse was moved off the ward while the complaint was investigated and dealt with, and as a result of stress was off sick for a long time. This event displays very clearly how patient manipulation, using the complaints system, can result in anger and recriminations between front-line staff and their managers who have the responsibility to investigate fairly and equitably any complaints.

Some nurses expressed understanding of the managers' point of view, giving reasons why they may be oversensitive and unrealistic. Firstly, the high political profile of the High Security Hospitals and their inmates, engendering a sense that everything the managers do is potentially open to public scrutiny and criticism. Thus one nurse could comment about a patient that 'we felt that, the management were listening to him, 'cos they were frightened about what was going to happen in the Press, 'cos of his contact with an MP'. Secondly, managers themselves are afraid of what might happen to them if they do not handle a complaint with absolute objectivity and total adherence to the rules of the process. Hence another nurse reported that the 'management are too frightened to say no to any of the people with personality disorder, because then they start suing or making letters of complaint, which are sometimes upheld'. Thirdly, some nurses recognized that it is difficult for managers to tell at one remove, without knowing in depth the nurse and patient concerned, what is a serious and what is a truly trivial complaint. Lastly, some of the nurses knew that the patient abuse and nursing malpractice of the past (covered in several inquiry reports) made the allegations of patients easier to believe, and they were thus taken more seriously. The nurses who acknowledged the pressures on managers were more able to tolerate the stressful official complaints procedure, seeing it as necessary to prevent patients becoming 'disempowered', 'submissive' or 'cowed' as they had been in the recent past.

For those staff who had no appreciation of the external forces within which managers had to work, the complaints process as endured or as observed in its mastication of other nurses, engendered hostility towards, and alienation from, managers. Staff were left feeling disappointed, under the impression that PD patients 'run the management', and with a strong negative evaluation of managers in general: *And we have found in the past that when you deal with an incident to do with a PD, and before you know it you have got management crawling all over you, with a complaint that this chap has made which is totally untrue.*

To a great extent, patients' manipulation of managers has been covered elsewhere, where it was described how PD patients wield influence outside the hospital, open gaps in policy, and interfere in the nursing staff hierarchy in order to get what they want. Several examples were given by nurses of how PD patients sought to subvert senior nurses' trust and confidence in their staff. These examples are illuminating and are quoted in full:

The night charge had come on the ward and he sat in the night station with us, and he was going, this patient at eleven-o-clock – to walk to his side room with a cigarette. We said to him 'you can't go down there smoking at eleven-o-clock'. And he said, 'you didn't stop me last night'. And we said 'we did, we stop you every night'. And he said, 'no you didn't, I come down here half past eleven smoking, you didn't stop me'. And then the night manager's there, and that's all it was, the night manager was there. So because we pulled him up, he thought I'll get one up on you, I'll tell him this. When he went the night manager he said 'is that right then, are you doing that just because I'm here or what?' And we said 'You weigh it up. Do we?' And he said 'well no, I don't think so'.

Well, for an example, like one in particular at the moment, she's on medica-tion. And she's had all her PRN [medication prescribed and given at the nurses discretion], *and she come up to me and said 'oh, can I have my PRN?' I said, 'no you've had it'. 'Oh please I need it, I need it, I need it.' I said 'I'm sorry but you've had it, right'. 'Oh go on just let me have a little bit, I won't tell any-body, go on.' You know what I mean? This sort of thing, this is just an example 'cos it happened to me only two nights ago in fact. I said, 'I'm sorry I'm not going to do it.' 'I'm going to see* [name of ward manager deleted] *about you in the morning.'... She said 'I'm going to report you and say that you've given me the wrong medication', trying to blackmail me right? So of course, of course I've had a chat to her about it, discussed it with her, saw* [name of ward manager deleted] *in the morning, and said 'look I'm sorry, this is what she is saying', you know and hopefully* [name of ward manager deleted] *believes me and not the patient.*

The interesting point to observe here is that it is absolutely impossible for the manager to know what the truth of the issue is, as it is the manager's role to ensure that staff fulfil their duties properly, and everybody knows that employees do on occasion break rules or seek to cut corners. The manager must choose either to trust the staff or the patient, and even if he or she elect to do the former, the patient has sown a seed of doubt, and undermined the organizational cohesion. The only partial remedy for this situation is for the manager to know the staff and their capabilities well, and the patients' capabilities equally well.

Any hierarchical system has the capacity to generate and maintain mis-trust and cynicism. The presence of PD patients within the High Security Hospitals exacerbates and multiplies this problem because of: the manipula-tive subversion of the hierarchy by patients; the harsh and hypersensitive complaints system which is not fully understood by staff; and the mirroring of PD sensitivity to criticism by nurses and managers. These three conditions and their associated problems inevitably poison relationships between nurses and their managers.

Thus the picture that emerges from the remainder of the data on manage-ment is of managers being disparaged and treated with suspicion by nurses who are part of the ward-based team. *We don't see the patients as an adversary, we're here to look after them, to the best we can, but we say the adversary is the management, you know. They're not on our side, that's my opinion, quite a number of guys' opinion.* Thus most of the positive comments about managers providing advice and guidance mention the excellent support from ward managers and team leaders, saying things like 'they've always been there for us' and 'they're quite supportive, helpful, if you are experiencing problems with a particular client . . . they can help you overcome that'. The team leaders and ward managers talk about receiving advice and support from nurses on other wards at their own level, not from their managers, saying things like 'I'm comfortable with contacting other wards and asking them how they dealt with certain issues'. Nobody interviewed spoke of middle managers giving a clinical lead, and some specifically ruled them out as sources of expertise, saying 'the only advice you get is from your direct colleagues on the ward'.

The gap between nurses and their non-ward-based managers is nowhere more evident than here. The keenest, most expert ward managers are the ones who are able to win promotion to middle management grades. Yet it appears that, the moment they obtain such a position, their clinical advice becomes worthless because of the antipathy between the two groups. Thus the ward managers are left in a position of self-imposed isolation, giving clinical leadership to all below them, but only willing to accept it from their peers.

This credibility gap is further widened if managers fail to have a physical profile on the ward, 'never come inside the ward', 'wouldn't know where [name of ward deleted] is, if they walked into the door', 'always off dealing with something' or at a 'meeting'. The sense that managers do not face the same dangers of serious physical assault from patients is keenly felt by nurses, especially when new difficult policies which are likely to put staff in danger are brought out by managers. When managers do have a presence, and do get involved, this is highly valued by staff and increases their credibility. In the wake of the Fallon Inquiry, because of fears about the spread of pornography, patients had their videos removed. Those managers who came and stood on the front line during that inflammable process, and 'took the flak off the patient' rose in the respect of the staff.

Finally, the formation of mutual trust between nurses and their managers has not been aided by frequent changes, restructuring and reorganization. Staff complained that 'in the last ten years, they've have had three or four different managements here' or a 'succession of managers'. So changeable was the situation that some found it a source of black humour: 'this is Ashworth, (chuckles) the management changes day to day'.

The splitting of the two groups of staff, partly created by PD behaviour, is evidenced in a number of additional ways. Nurses criticize the policies made or not made by the managers; they feel the managers do not really understand the difficulties of dealing with PD patients and therefore make unrealistic plans. They consider that managers are more likely to back patients than staff if there is any conflict; that they are only interested in looking after themselves; that they do not listen to nurses; and do not offer sufficient support and sympathy to nurses following violent incidents. In other words, the mistrust and lack of confidence between nurses and their managers saps morale, makes the organization dysfunctional, and handicaps it with internal conflicts.

Multidisciplinary teamwork

Although nurses were not asked any specific questions about medical staff and multidisciplinary teamwork, they did make quite a number of comments, usually in the course of making replies about treatability and treatment. These comments were both positive and negative, depending upon the individual nurse's past experiences and current perspectives of this parallel discipline. From this material it is possible to formulate a description of what is, from the psychiatric nurse's point of view, the best way for psychiatrists to operate in order to facilitate the care and treatment of PD patients.

The authority of doctors over admission, treatment, leave, and discharge was widely acknowledged, assumed and highly valued in the nurses' comments. At its best, the way this was translated into action was by wide-ranging and open discussion within the multidisciplinary team, followed by the consultant having the final say: *But it will go to the clinical team meeting, and others will say, on clinical grounds the RMO* [Responsible Medical Officer], *and then that will go up to Dr N to actually sign in the end.* At its worst, nurses sometimes felt publicly humiliated by the rejection of their views: *You sit in CTMs* [Care Team Meetings] *and the doc, the medical staff here I think, are appalling, I've actually sat through a CTM and had a doctor tell me more or less that my opinion was irrelevant.* Or by their exclusion from the provision of psychological treatments: *You know this, from what I can see, the majority is like; they go on these group sessions with the psychiatrist and that. I think there should be more input from the nursing staff.*

Nurses saw the medical staff as a source of expertise and education, with many expressing the view that they had learned a great deal about personality disorder in this way. This dynamic had the added benefit of enhancing nurses' respect for medical leadership, and some spoke of their medical colleagues with deeply felt regard. Because of their role and authority, doctors have the capacity to galvanize the entire clinical team into coherent, directed action, and nurses looked to them for this type of leadership. One nurse spoke of a 'young, vibrant, forward thinking doctor' who 'gave us direction'. Within this context of medical leadership, divided opinion among doctors about the treatability of PD was problematic for nurses. They sought to take a lead from medical staff but clearly could not do so easily on this particular issue. Given their leadership position, doctors could therefore exert a dramatic influence upon the morale of the team. This worked both ways. If they were negative about the prospects of therapeutic improvement in PD patients, this dampened enthusiasm among the nurses, but a positive approach generated energy in the team.

The support that can be given by medical staff to nurses was extremely highly valued, and many saw it as crucial to daily patient management on the ward. Psychiatrists gave this support by upholding the ward rules and patient care strategies put into operation by the nurses. This was most noticeable when it was absent. When doctors countermanded, in an arbitrary manner, the day-to-day decisions made by nurses, without conference or consultation, the nurses were placed in an impossible situation and their authority to control events on the ward undermined. Ways in which psychiatrists can support nurses are: by having a real presence on the ward, visiting patients frequently and conferring with the nurses; giving verbal support to the whole hospital patient care system; using their greater authority to persuade patients to comply with nursing care strategies; and adequately medicating violent patients so as to prevent injuries to nurses.

In the eyes of nurses, the medical staff must also fulfil their responsibilities to the multidisciplinary team by resisting the manipulative strategies of patients. PD patients deliberately seek to disempower the nurses by inveigling medical staff to change the ward rules: *The guys who were constantly abusing the catalogues would be one. The guys who, they'd only tell you, right I'll give the doctors the right answers, you lot can go fuck yourself, you know I don't have to do it, the doctor will come in and sort us out. They were right. If they had a problem with the way we ran the ward, they went and saw the doctors and the doctors – 'Did we really need to do that?'* Other ways in which patients sought to manipulate medical staff were: by persuading them to prescribe desired medications; swaying them to preferentially accept their suggestions so as to become a leader in the informal patient hierarchy; misleading them about their symptoms in order to get a desired diagnosis; demanding their time and attention; and causing splits and disagreements between nurses and doctors by only agreeing to talk to the latter.

Key events can shape the nursing teams' views of individual psychiatrists, powerfully impacting upon the subsequent teamwork and working relationships. Nurses described two of these events. In the first a doctor came to the aid of a nurse who was being held hostage, resulting in strong cross-disciplinary commitment and bonding: *And our RMO was N who is the most, I describe as a woman with balls. She's got guts, she's got grit for want of a better word, she's a classy bird that one, woman. No, she's all right, she's all right, she come up trumps, she stood up there four hours talking for England. Communication's the name of the game and she done it well, I respect millions for her, she done well.* In the second instance, a doctor behaved in what nurses considered to be an inappropriate manner towards a patient, bringing her a present of videotapes in order to persuade her to accept a depot injection: *Me personally, I've got that in the back of my mind and I'm thinking 'I know you're a wally' and that's how I'm going to think of him. It'll take a lot now for me to change my opinion of him for doing that.*

To summarize, what nurses look for in psychiatrists are that they should:

- give a clear, consistent, enthusiastic and committed lead to treatment content, and express optimism about eventual therapeutic progress;
- allow and facilitate nurses taking a role in psychological treatment;
- be present on the ward frequently, talking and listening to both nurses and patients;
- confer with the nurses and listen respectfully to their views before taking decisions;
- uphold the ward rules with patients, be aware of patients' manipulation and refuse to go along with it;
- educate the nurses in the course of their daily clinical work;
- show concern and support for nurses in their task of patient management, do what is possible to assist in the resolution of the problems that they face.

Nurses also perceive psychologists as having a very significant contribution to make in the treatment of PD patients, with some seeing them as the sole agents of psychological treatment, and others commenting on the scarcity of psychologists and the need for more input. Nurses value psychologists for their one-to-one work with patients around their index offence, for their leadership of therapeutic groups, especially those for sex offenders, and for their ability to carry out cognitive-behavioural interventions with PD patients. Psychologists are also perceived as an important source of education, learning and supervision. Nurses mentioned their contribution to specialist PD induction courses at Rampton Hospital, while others valued the things they had learned from their contributions to multidisciplinary team meetings. One nurse was lucky enough to have received individual clinical supervision from a psychologist and declared this to be very helpful.

They are looked upon as experts, and nurses sought their answers to questions of current research findings, treatment approaches, and ethical issues. Nurses also spoke approvingly about the opportunities they had to work with psychologists as co-therapists in the running of groups. The responsibility psychologists had had in the founding of the specialist PD services at Rampton and Ashworth was also mentioned and acknowledged by the nurses.

All in all, psychologists and their input were well respected. However, this is not to say that there were not areas of conflict. The use of High Security Hospitals for training psychologists is seen as damaging to patients, in that at the end of their placement period the patient whom they have been working with is either 'dropped' (i.e. receives no further individual therapy) or has to start again with another worker. Their transient presence on the ward as students, or contributors to multidisciplinary meetings, or just as visitors to the ward, caused some nurses to refer to them as 'tourists'. When psychologists fail to communicate and liaise with nursing staff, this is found to be offensive and to cause difficulties with patients. Two types of problem were mentioned in this respect. Firstly, the patient can be upset after an individual therapy session, and nurses have difficulty dealing with this as they are not aware of what caused the problem. More acutely, however, the failure to communicate makes nurses feel excluded, undervalued and 'quite worthless'. There is a parallel here between this and the catastrophic feelings associated with 'being undermined' by managers.

Social workers received less comment in these interviews, and the few comments that were passed were usually in relation to dealing with patients' relatives and families. No consistent picture emerges of working relationships between nurses and social workers. Their role in liaising with patients' relatives is valued, but nurses also criticize them on a variety of grounds. They are said to have too rosy a view of patients and a stereotyped negative attitude to nurses: *But if you listen to some of the social workers here, you would think they were Snow White followed by the demon Seven Dwarfs – that being the staff!* Like the psychologists and doctors, their occasional failure to communicate with the ward nurses caused difficulties in managing patients, and hence some conflict.

Thus with all three disciplines, conflict can be created with nurses by poor communication and by the manipulative behaviour of PD patients. That conflict corrodes multidisciplinary teamwork, and probably negatively affects the care given to some patients.

Training and education for working with PD patients

In many ways the interviews demonstrated a need for training staff in working with PD patients. One of the self-management mechanisms that assisted nurses in maintaining a positive attitude was to develop a psychological understanding of difficult patient behaviour. Yet many aspects of the interviews showed that, for some nurses, such understanding was poor or absent.

Take, for example, manipulation. Strikingly few nurses gave any motivational explanation as to why PD patients behaved in this way. There were a few mentions of the 'dynamics' of manipulation, but these were made without any further explanation. Instead the behaviour was labelled and contained, rather than understood. When nurses did offer interpretations, these were rudimentary rather than psychologically sophisticated. One nurse suggested that manipulation was a survival strategy learned during childhood – becoming 'streetwise' and learning that 'they can get things by manipulating, by threatening, and becoming the bullyboy' had become an ingrained and uncontrollable habit by adulthood. Another explained that, in her view, the patients' manipulation usually had some kind of moral logic, in that it was an attempt to express anger about some perceived slight or trespass, or to exact some form of revenge. Most offered no explanation or interpretation at all.

Views of self-harm were not quite as rudimentary, but were still not very articulate. There are many alternative explanations of self-injury that do not invoke manipulative bullying in any form. Not all of these were mentioned by nurses, and those that were were not well or confidently expressed. Points made touched on self-harm being:

- A natural means of emotional expression outside of the person's control, equivalent to howling, shouting, screaming, wailing or crying. Such expressions can be supplemented but not substituted by verbal expression. As with other natural impulses – for example, expressions of naked, raw emotion – self-injury may be, to a degree on some occasions, facilitated or inhibited by the person and those around them.
- An institutional behaviour, prevalent in deprived environments with low stimulation. Self-injury may be a stimulant, removing emotional boredom, and equivalent to head banging, rocking, picking and plucking at the body.
- A tension-relieving device, alleviating strong and overwhelming negative feelings towards or about oneself. Or distracting one's own attention from such feelings, via the provision of a strong alternative focus for consciousness, blocking negative thoughts and emotions. Or cancelling them through self-punishment.
- A way of remedying dissociative states, where one feels unreal, alienated, divorced from the world and one's body.
- A means of communicating the reality and intensity of distress, when others appear not to understand or fully comprehend the profound depth of one's desolation.

The staff did not show a high awareness of the literature about self-harm and its potential underlying psychological explanations. As a result, those psychological explanations were not available to them in their daily interactions with patients, and they were probably more likely to fall back on their natural angry reactions.

As in other areas, nurses did little theorizing about the underlying, long-term causes of patient violence. A few nurses linked the violence of patients to their past experience of abuse: *Pressures through childhood that have made them adapt, have to adapt to society in a sort of very aggressive way because that's the environment that they have been brought up in.* Others saw it as evidencing long-term difficulty with anyone in a position of authority, or as a consequence of the nurses holding them imprisoned within the hospital or representing the society that kept them there. Mostly, nurses appeared to take violence from PD patients as a 'given', a natural expression of the pathology of the condition. A few said this explicitly, but most demonstrated this view by an unquestioning acceptance of the reality of aggressive behaviour from this patient group: *You know, aggression can be a common expression from somebody suffering from a PD.*

Similarly many nurses' comments on the reasons for patients' complaints showed a lack of psychological understanding. Instead they appeared to think concretely and superficially about patient motivations in making complaints. The power and intensity of the nurse–patient relationship did not seem to be appreciated, and psychological interpretations or understandings of patient criticism and complaints were rare. Yet potential psychological explanations are not hard to find, even at the level of the mundane. Anybody who is imprisoned and herded into a faceless institution will seek to maximize some control over the situation, to find an outlet to achieve a sense of freedom, and will try to express his or her individuality and self-worth. Given that so many PD patients may have gnawing feelings of worthlessness and powerlessness, covered with a fragile veneer of self-respect, the use of the complaints procedure to assert their own value is unsurprising. In addition, given PD patients' paranoia and hypersensitivity to criticism, it is likely that they will perceive a dismissive attitude in staff even when it is not present. Thus, in their eyes the complaint they are making (or the revenge they are taking) may be comprehensible and justifiable.

Complaints made in response to frustration may represent patients' need for affirmation, coupled with plummeting bad feelings about themselves when something is refused. The trivial thing they are denied may have great symbolic weight in their mind, and their scale of values be entirely different from the neutral observer. To the continuously hurting, fragile, paranoid person a refusal may symbolize every previous occasion in which he was dismissed as a worthwhile person, and every attempt to stamp him into the ground. Therefore he fights back, tooth and nail, with great anger and emotion, as a matter of psychological survival. The false allegation is perhaps more difficult to comprehend. Here there is no easily recognizable, overt trigger. Yet it still may not be power the patient seeks *per se*; it may be an expression of primitive anger, hatred and rage – a need to punish someone else, perhaps in response to an imagined slight, or perhaps because of a threatened intimacy that arouses strong anxiety. More outstanding is the nurses' complete failure to understand why patients may complain of assault when they have only been restrained. It takes but little empathetic thought to realize that the perceptions and the emotional response to being restrained of somebody who has been seriously physically abused as a child are going to be extreme. Thus patients may experience flashbacks during such high-stress, high-fear situations, and may genuinely believe that they have yet again been brutalized and assaulted.

Perhaps part of the reason nurses find it hard to think about these patient behaviours with psychological understanding is that their own reactions are also strongly emotional. On these occasions nurses can feel betrayed, disappointed and let down by the patients they are trying to help and care for. In addition, their sense of control over events is threatened in an environment in which it is very important that it be maintained – for their own safety and that of their colleagues and the general public. Finally, if the complaint is about a nurse as an individual, then that person's livelihood and future career are threatened. However, many nurses clearly lacked any theoretical framework or educational structure that would enable them to view the complaining behaviour of PD patients in a psychological context that made it both explicable and manageable.

There were three possible sources of training for nurses: basic professional education; the induction course upon taking up a post within a High Security Hospital; post-basic courses completed while working there. The interviews revealed that in respect of the care and treatment of PD patients, all were problematic in one way or another.

Views of the interviewees on their basic nurse training were quite varied. The most common refrain was that they had received very little in the way of course content on PD. Others felt that they had acquired some knowledge and/or skills pertaining to PD, but an equal number felt completely unprepared for the type of problems and issues they faced in PD care in the High Security Hospitals. Perhaps this is not surprising, as these hospitals are unique environments, and the patients are qualitatively different from those encountered in general psychiatric settings. A few nurses reported that their basic training had imbued them with negative attitudes towards PD: specifically that PD was an untreatable condition. However, more referred to the fact that basic training had been a period in their lives when they had acquired high ethical values and commitments to the care of the mentally ill which were directly applicable to the care of PD patients: for example, 'client choice' and 'respecting individuals'. The questionnaire survey showed that nursing grade was associated with overall attitude to PD, with lower grades (i.e. unqualified staff) having more negative attitudes. This may imply that, in general, nurse training contributes to positive attitudes to PD.

Overall, the induction courses available were not evaluated very positively. Some staff had difficulty in commenting on the induction course because they had started so long ago they could hardly remember it. Of those who could give a clear evaluation, the largest group said that it was of little value in relation to PD. Generally it was viewed to be too short (lasting only a week or two) with no content on PD patient care. Some responses were disparaging and dismissive, saying the induction was 'a complete waste of time', 'crap', 'the most boring week of my life' or 'rubbish'. The content on security issues, control and restraint training, resuscitation, fires, was generally seen as valid, but insufficient in preparing nurses to confront the difficulties posed by PD patients. Those nurses who agreed that the induction was somewhat helpful also mentioned similar topics, but expressed more overall appreciation of their importance. Those expressing confidence in and satisfaction with the induction were in a minority. It was clear from the replies that many wards organized for themselves a supplementary induction for their new staff because of the perceived insufficiencies of the generic hospital induction, but this was mainly composed of giving new staff a period of time working with another nurse as mentor.

As a consequence of the content of the induction programme, many nurses felt completely unprepared to deal with the day-to-day care of PD patients.

They felt as if they had been 'thrown in at the deep end'. *Because you've got to cram so much into a week you just do not have time to take everything in, and you don't start really to know what you've let yourself in for till you actually walk on that ward. I know the first day . . . I was a nervous wreck, and I came through them gates, I didn't know what the hell I was to expect when I walked on that ward and to me I was terrified.* Others thought that this lack of preparation contributed to a high staff turnover, and remarked on the number of new staff who left very quickly after starting. In a striking statement of the realities of the situation, one nurse said: *Here, you can go from filling shelves on a supermarket and after a two-week induction to looking after a concentrated mass of murderers and killers and very dangerous people with very little adequate training.* This being said, the induction course does thoroughly cover the security aspects of the job, as other nurses commented. Nevertheless, there is a great deal more to surviving work with PD patients than this.

Respondents were classified into whether they had had no specialist post-basic training, some, or a substantial course. Criteria for a substantial course were a duration of at least one week, or a day release course spanning several months. The category of 'some training' included those who had attended occasional study days.

Substantive course attendees (20 per cent)   Most nurses in this category were from the Rampton PD unit. When that unit was first opened, all nurses received a specific and comprehensive induction course that was highly rated and appreciated by those nurses interviewed. Some specific courses were also available at Ashworth, although relatively few staff had managed to access them. The lowest number having attended a substantive course on PD was at Broadmoor Hospital. The main other course mentioned was the Forensic Mental Health Nursing diploma.

Those having received some training (21 per cent)   These encompassed study days on a variety of issues related to PD care, or were those who attended substantive courses on non-PD topics that covered some PD-specific material.

Not trained (54 per cent)   Most nurses in this category responded with a simple 'no' or 'none whatsoever' when asked if they had received any training on the care of PD, with some commenting that this type of course 'was practically non-existent'. These nurses remarked that they had learned how to care for PD patients by a process of watching others, and by trial and error. Most considered this to be both inefficient and dangerous, emphasizing the need for more systematic training initiatives, with one nurse advising others: *Get educated. Do anything you can, follow the courses . . . any course that's run, ward based, or over in the staff education centre, pertaining to PDs. Anything that goes into, anything about any drugs courses, anything that can teach you how to talk a patient down and back from a violent situation. Basically anything that you can get your hands on about PDs, do it. Wish I had.* Nurses working on PD units were more likely to have had some form of specific training, whether through odd study days or a substantive course. However, 41 per cent had still not had any specific training whatsoever.

It is difficult to view this situation as anything other than abysmal. The High Security Hospitals contain the most difficult PD patients in the country, and the staff that seek to manage them face tremendous problems on a day-to-day basis. Yet most staff are completely untrained in the care of PD patients. The generic induction provides little or nothing about PD care, and basic nurse training is patchy, with many graduating nurses having received little training about this patient group. Access to courses within the High Security Hospitals is obviously difficult for staff in post, given financial constraints, shortages of staff and the necessity to be on the wards. It is no wonder that the questionnaire survey revealed that only 1 in 4 nurses felt adequately trained to work with PD patients.

Clinical supervision

Clinical supervision is generally understood as requiring one-to-one meetings between a nurse and supervisor (not usually their line manager), on a regular basis, for the discussion of clinical nursing issues. It is held to have three functions (Hawkins and Shohet 1989, Proctor 1988):

Formative   Tthe development of skills through the presentation of clinical case material, discussion, brainstorming ideas and the giving of expert advice and instruction.

Normative   Maintaining accountability and high standards of practice through joint analysis of clinical casework and reflection upon what professional standards mean in application to individual cases and situations.

Restorative   Support of the supervisee as a person through examination of the impact clinical work is having, both personally and professionally.

Clinical supervision was introduced into psychiatric nursing practice during the 1980s, primarily among Community Psychiatric Nurses. There are several UK nursing champions of the cause of clinical supervision (Wilkin 1988, Cutcliffe and Proctor 1998, Butterworth *et al.* 1996, Power 1999) who advocate its wide implementation and use by psychiatric nurses. Although well accepted within community settings (although even there resistance to implementation has been noted by Wilkin *et al.* 1997), many have described structural and practical difficulties in its use within inpatient settings like the High Security Hospitals (Hughes and Morcom 1998).

Clinical supervision is most strongly established at Rampton Hospital, with 56 per cent of staff in regular supervisory meetings, as compared to 34 per cent at Ashworth and 23 per cent at Broadmoor. The higher the grade of staff, the more likely they were to be receiving regular supervision. Nursing assistants are the least likely to be receiving supervision, with several of them reporting in the interviews that it was only 'for qualified staff'. Not all staff even understood what clinical supervision meant: for example, one nurse asked 'doesn't that just mean that there's a qualified nurse within a certain distance?'

Being in receipt of supervision was very strongly associated with a positive overall attitude to PD. As with other findings in this cross-sectional study, it is impossible to be certain about the direction of causality. It is possible that the positive nurses were more likely to seek out or continue in clinical supervision. However, in the three hospitals covered by the study, one appeared to have implemented clinical supervision in a well-organized and thorough fashion, as over half the nurses received it on a regular basis. It is unlikely to be coincidental that the nurses in this hospital had the best overall attitude to PD. If we can assume that the three hospitals recruit nurses with the same general mix of overall attitude, then it seems likely that supervision is a significant ingredient in improving nurses' attitudes towards PD patients. This interpretation is further supported by the likelihood that nurses both learn and sharpen their self-management methods in clinical supervision, as this would clearly be an intrinsic part of the practice of clinical supervision in these settings. Lastly, what nurses have to say about the benefits of clinical supervision also supports this interpretation.

The forum of the clinical supervision meetings provided a protected space within which staff could 'off-load' their feelings, the stresses and strains of the job. These anxieties could be fears and worries about themselves or their patients, suppressed anger and frustration, or upset and distress regarding events that had taken place on the ward or what patients were saying. Nurses spoke of this as 'getting it off their shoulders' or 'having a good moan'. One female nurse described how a patient was talking of his sexual fantasies about her, and how she was able to tolerate this and use it therapeutically because in supervision she could release and share her emotional reactions. Another sense in which clinical supervision was found to be supportive was that it validated the nurses' feelings and reactions towards patients. Nurses felt that while they were 'on stage' practising their work, they had to display to patients and colleagues a persona of calm competence. However, in clinical supervision they had a place to take their real reactions where they would be accepted. The fact that time was available for that purpose helped nurses to feel less lonely.

Closely allied to the supportive function of clinical supervision, with its facilitation and validation of nurses' emotional expression, is the analysis of those emotions and responses to patients with a consequent growth in self-awareness. In clinical supervision sessions nurses learned to question and examine their emotional reactions to patients, and ask themselves why they were reacting in these particular ways. With the help of their supervisors they were able to find answers to these questions that assisted them in responding appropriately to the demands made upon them by difficult PD patients. One nurse called this supervisory process 'challenging yourself', and another reported how he had been enabled to locate some of the sources of his angry reactions towards a patient, and had learned to question himself and his motivations to a much greater degree.

Patient awareness was the other side of the coin. Clinical supervision was a time when nurses could reflect not just upon their reactions to patients, but also on the ways patients were behaving towards them. Sometimes this meant a growing recognition of how patients were evoking emotional reactions in the nurse: *And also for nurses to recognize that they have an effect on you, to recognize that they do often make you feel the way that they feel, transfer everything onto you. And I think that's where clinical supervision is essential.* At other times it meant achieving an awareness as to how patients might be seeking to manipulate the nurse: *They can actually gradually think very carefully about bringing you down to a person that they can control in some way . . . and you have to be on your guard and you've got to be alert to, you know, how some of these patents can do this over a period of time. Particularly, you know, if you're working quite closely with them on a daily basis and with their emotions. This is . . . this comes back to supervision again and why supervision is so important.* Another nurse described how she had slipped into a pattern of responding to a patient's distress and threats by regularly staying on after her shift to discuss these with the patient, and had not realized the existence of this pattern until it was identified in supervision. So for these nurses clinical supervision was helpful in that it kept them aware of appropriate boundaries to their behaviour, preventing them from 'being sucked in' or manipulated, by providing them with objective feedback on what they were doing.

Several nurses reported that developing expertise was for them the main function of clinical supervision. They took clinical dilemmas, cases and situations to their supervisor, and looked for expert advice or help with the generation of new ideas and nursing strategies. *I tend to take not so much generic issues like dealing with personality disorder, but dealing with particular situations I don't know, such as conflict management or something, 'well this is what I did to de-escalate things, what do you think? Could I've done it a different way?'* As a consequence, nurses believed that their practice of psychiatric nursing had improved through the supervision process.

If it can be concluded that clinical supervision does contribute to the development and maintenance of a positive attitude to PD patients, then this carries the implication that the establishment and support of clinical supervisory systems should be a priority for those who care for PD patients as a regular part of their work. Furthermore, the efficacy of clinical supervision within PD care settings could be enhanced by a modicum of agenda setting by the supervisor, based around the beliefs and self-management methods that this research has revealed are associated with positive attitudes.

Moreover, this finding, that clinical supervision is associated with positive nurse attitudes to PD, is one further pebble in the growing pile of evidence on the general value and efficacy of clinical supervision for nurses. Other studies have shown that nurses report benefits from undertaking regular clinical supervision (Bowles and Young 1999, Paunonen 1991, Severinsson and Hallberg 1996). To date, no study has been undertaken that seeks to evaluate the impact upon patients themselves. However, as the evidence grows, it becomes harder to resist the conclusion that clinical supervision does benefit patient care.

Summary

The behaviour of PD patients exacerbates conflict that ricochets through the hospital system, widening divisions and sowing distrust between staff and their managers, and between the different professions in the psychiatric multidisciplinary team. Emotions are heightened by the pressures exerted by patients through all six forms of manipulative behaviour (which threaten the life, limb, employment security and reputation of staff), and possibly through the sensitization of nurses to threats to their self-esteem from continuous contact with PD patients. Holding this together while under the constantly scrutinizing gaze of the media, professional bodies, Mental Health Act commission, etc., cannot be an easy task, especially when one form of manipulative behaviour – capitalizing – directly seeks to exploit any external hierarchy or power source like these. In order to overcome these problems the organization as a whole needs to invest great efforts in maintaining open communication and good liaison between all subgroups, whether they be disciplinary or hierarchically based.

Furthermore, there are two main ways in which the organization can promote positive attitudes to PD patients: (1) the provision of training that will give staff the knowledge, skills and psychological understanding that underpin positive attitudes to PD; and (2) the implementation of structures of regular clinical supervision for staff, so that they can be supported, emotionally validated, grow in patient and self-awareness, and develop their expertise.

6   Effects and impacts

The mechanisms behind positive attitudes have now been thoroughly described. Staff who enjoyed working with PD patients and felt secure, accepting, purposeful and enthusiastic, tended to hold different beliefs about PD and its treatment and have different moral commitments, interpersonal skills, ways of managing their own emotions, etc., than those nurses who found the tasks more demanding. Moreover, the hospital culture within which they worked had a strong impact, either to enable or hinder that positive attitude among staff. Those organizations that provided training and clinical supervision, and which overcame the exacerbation of conflict produced by PD patients between hierarchical and disciplinary divisions, provided a cultural environment within which positive attitudes could flourish.

However, it would be a mistake to think that having a positive attitude to working with PD patients was simply a matter of feeling good about work. Rather the holding of positive or negative attitudes could be highly consequential, and not just for the behaviour of nurses within the work environment, but also for the impact that work had upon their personal lives and feelings of well-being outside of the hospital. That impact could be profound and quite shocking, indicating that, for some staff, working with PD patients could be psychologically and socially corrosive. For others it could lead to definite gains in personal development. In this chapter the effects and impacts of these positive and negative attitudes will be detailed.

The following sections seek to lay out exactly the effects of a positive or negative attitude, as evidenced by what the interviewees said, mainly about their own behaviour and responses to patients. For ease of description, the two attitudes have been treated as representing two different categories of nurse. However, it is important to realize that although the impacts described below are associated, sometimes very strongly, with attitude, the correlations are not perfect. It is even more important to realize that few staff fit perfectly into being uniformly representative of either category. Attitudes to PD followed the normal bell-shaped distribution curve – that is, there were few people at extreme poles, with more in the middle with a rather mixed attitude to PD, some leaning one way and some the other.

This chapter will also specifically explore the relationship between attitudes to PD and the maintenance of control and order on the wards, expressed by nurses as 'structure'. Positive nurses did have a different view on this, but not because they were less concerned with security than the negative nurses; nor were they necessarily more naïve or soft touches for the manipulative PD patient. It would be all too easy to dichotomize nurses in an unhelpful way by suggesting that nurses with a positive attitude are caring and good, but soft, naïve and prone to exploitation by patients; whereas it could be argued that nurses with a negative attitude were cynical, but strong, realistic and much more likely to maintain security. This simplistic picture, however, is not sustained by the interviews. Firstly, nurses did not fall into completely different groups since attitudes were normally distributed. Secondly, the positive nurses were no less concerned with safety and security than the negative nurses. However, they did seek to create an effective structure in a different way. The *modus operandi* that was actually better at keeping order was not a question within the scope of this study, but remains a priority for future research. There are, however, some preliminary indications that the methods more frequently advocated by those with a negative attitude were ineffective, or ineffectively applied by those nurses.

Negative nursing in a negative organization

All nurses working with PD patients in the High Security Hospitals had to find ways to come to terms emotionally with the reality of patients' index offences. Those staff who could not find a way to do this left the service very quickly. Those who stayed found that they had to suppress thoughts about the crimes that patients had committed. The consequences of not doing so were seen as both internal and external. Some staff suggested that if they did not suppress these thoughts, if they 'came on duty thinking evil things all the time', then their own mental health would suffer (*it would blow your head, wouldn't it?*). Externally, many nurses realized that it would be impossible to have a conversation with or relate to patients unless the crime was ignored: *To be able to relate to them, to be able to talk to them, you have to put behind, you know, to one side, not so much behind but more to one side, the fact that this man has raped and killed, you know, a five-year-old girl. It would be very difficult if that was at the forefront of your mind to actually have a conversation with somebody.* Not only can general social intercourse be handicapped, perceiving the right way to treat patients therapeutically could be obscured by the angry emotions raised when thinking about the patients' criminal offences: *Because I believe that it's not an objective manner of describing* [an] *individual, and that will not allow us to get to the heart of the treatment issues.* Thus from a purely practical and pragmatic point of view the nurses were motivated to ignore or repress thoughts about the patients' index offences.

The positive nurses had a range of beliefs, moral commitments and self-management methods that allowed and justified the setting aside of angry thoughts about index offences. The negative nurses tended not to have recourse to these methods. As a consequence, out of practical necessity they suppressed these thoughts, or their angry feelings found expression in the terminology of evil: patients were regarded as, and called, bad, evil, or monstrous. This anger could have a number of further outcomes. In some cases patients were simply avoided, the nurses concerned would not interact with those who had done things that they were unable to tolerate. In other cases, nurses could pass on their views, and some patients started to think of themselves as bad and evil – a factor that hindered treatment and progress through a reinforcement of their pathology (*it just reinforces their whole negative feeling about themselves and everybody else*). Finally, these angry feelings could result in staff mirroring of PD behaviour. One nurse gave the example of a patient who came to the ward office door to ask for something, and one staff member said to another, 'He's an evil bastard, let him wait.' The nurse relating this tale then went on to comment 'who's the more personality disordered, some of the staff or the patients?', thus recognizing that in their apparently righteous anger towards the patients who have committed horrible crimes, nurses start to mirror PD behaviour, albeit in a minor form.

Being the butt of sustained verbal abuse, hostility, criticisms and threats was a difficult situation for staff. Such was the degree of pressure that they could come close, entirely naturally, to losing their temper and responding emotionally. The positive nurses had a whole series of ways to prevent this, ways to protect themselves from their own natural responses, including giving objective, unemotional feedback to the patients concerned, about the impact of their behaviour, and using the situation as an opportunity for therapeutic learning. The negative attitude nurses tended not to realize that this was an option. Instead they believed that they could do nothing, with 'not respond', 'go blank', 'just walk away', 'shut yourself down', 'just stand there and take it', being some of the responses described. This nurse did not realize that there was another option, and only the realities of the complaints procedures held his temper in check: *Angry at times because I want to tell them people what I think of them, you know, it's putting me in that situation but things hold me back because you have to be so aware of whatever we say to these people because we could be, impending investigation, management are going to be on your back or whatever you say is wrong as far as I am concerned, I mean I am straight John Bull, I want to tell them how I feel about what they put me under, without it going any further, the incident stops there, you know, if somebody is abusive, verbally abusive towards me, then I want to stand up for myself.* He believed that there was nothing he could say which would not result in a complaint and investigation.

Not all nurses took the option of withdrawing from patients and not responding at all. One advanced the argument that the whole nursing team had to take a consistent line on verbal abuse by patients, and that if the team at all times refused to accept it from patients then they would no longer behave in that fashion: *So you have to have a group of staff that will sit down together and discuss and say, well, hang on – this behaviour we are not going to accept. Across the board we are not going to accept it. And that's the response you give to the patient. And it is amazing because it does work. The patients do find out that, if they're going to come up to you with that attitude, then they are not going to get anywhere.* In short this nurse recommended that patients be sent away, that the nurses should say this behaviour is unacceptable, and that demands made in this way were not to be met. The downside of this strategy is that it does not provide the role modelling that honest, open feedback does, nor does it seem realistic that a ward full of PD patients in a secure hospital can be made to totally desist from verbal abuse. There also seems to be a possibility of its being carried out by nurses in an angry and hostile manner, and feel quite punitive to the patient, for the same nurse went on to say, with some apparent satisfaction: *They are not even going to get a toilet roll for the toilet, because if you are going to swear at me, I don't want to know, I am not listening.*

This hostility from negative attitude nurses leaks in other ways. For example, in relation to the control of aggressive and other disruptive behaviour, sanctions and 'consequences' were more frequently mentioned by those with a negative attitude. These sanctions included restrictions on: ground parole; social activities and trips; access to personal property (e.g. TV or video); purchasing goods; transfer to a less desirable or more restrictive ward; access to one's own room; recording an incident in notes leading to longer stay in hospital; 'D' notice (incident record with similar effect); avoidance by nurses; seclusion; loss of home visits. These nurses viewed such sanctions, if clearly defined and declared to the patients in advance, as ways of inducing self-control and as limitations upon aggressive behaviour. Nurses described using these sanctions by neutrally reminding the patient when an aggressive incident was developing as to what can happen as a consequence. Statements about the need for such sanctions were often coupled with crude behaviouristic judgements about the need for PD patients to 'learn'. The anger of negative attitude nurses was also linked to the way in which they construed PD patients to be cognitively competent. They were viewed as being fully aware of what they did and therefore fully responsible. Thus the angry response of staff could be seen as justifiable.

It seems likely, therefore, that negative attitudes represent, to some degree, self-confirming and self-fulfilling prophesies. PD patients are extremely sensitive to criticism or disrespect, and it may be because they have a very fragile sense of self-esteem that they are driven to defend strongly, or because they have paranoid personality features and over-interpret the others' actions as hostile. Either way, they are likely to sense very quickly any anger or rejection, even when the nurses seek to hide their inner feelings. Their response would be more anger, more abuse, more complaints, and a lower valuation of nurses. The patients will also feel betrayed and let down by professionals who are ostensibly there to give them therapeutic care and help. This in turn seems likely to lead to more manipulation, more pathological behaviour, etc., thus confirming the negative and rejecting attitudes of the members of staff and strengthening their conclusion that PD patients can't be trusted. What is more, although there is no logical connection, the interviews demonstrated that experience of difficult patient behaviour (manipulation, let down, violence) could directly erode nurses' belief in treatability, leading to a more generalized sense of pessimism and futility.

Undergoing severe disappointments appeared to be intrinsic to the experience of looking after PD patients. These 'let down' experiences could be so emotionally shocking that the nurses were left feeling slightly bewildered, as if the ground had been taken from under their feet and they needed to re-evaluate their past interactions with the patients concerned: *It makes you angry, frustrated, it might be an attack from a patient that you built a relationship up with, and just totally unprovoked and from behind and it, it's confusing I would say, it confuses you.* If they failed to reach an understanding of the patients' behaviour, they could lapse into the global, negative, angry stereotyping of PD patients as completely untrustworthy. This is expressed by many nurses in the interviews in their recommendations 'never' to trust a PD patient, usually coupled with accounts of how they had been 'caught out' in the past. For example, one nurse explained how a patient, with whom he thought he had a good relationship, had made false allegations about him. Similarly, another nurse related a collapse of trust following the events that resulted in the Fallon inquiry: *You know PDs were all nice and friendly and yet they were doing things behind our backs that they shouldn't have been doing and we trusted them, . . . It blew up in our faces so you know, then you tend to think well no that won't happen again. We won't trust them again.* Alternatively or additionally, nurses can get angry with and reject patients who disappoint them in these ways. More than 1 in 5 of the interviewed nurses avowed that PD patients should either not be trusted at all, or be trusted with extreme caution. These recommendations were coupled, in some cases, with accounts of 'let down' experiences, or other tales of betrayal of nurse confidence. There was a weak association between those who made these assertions and an overall negative stance towards PD care. Many of these statements were either very blunt, or declared as lessons learned at high personal cost: *Don't trust them as far as you can throw them. Because they will get one over on you if they can. If they possibly can, they'll get one over on you. So. And make you look foolish and possibly make you lose your job.* These experiences engendered a sense of futility in some nurses: a few gave up the struggle, having become so disillusioned from such experiences that they left the forensic psychiatric services, or left nursing completely. *You can build up this good rapport with them, and okay you're always aware they can turn, but then maybe the next day they will attack you, they will verbally abuse you, they will throw something at you, they will do something and you think, God, why do I bother? And that is always there, you think, God, I am wasting my time, and that is hard.*

It can be noted here that in these settings a social engine naturally promotes cynical attitudes among staff. Nurses are concerned about how they appear in the eyes of their colleagues. Of course they do not want to be manipulated by a patient because it will have a negative outcome for staff and patient alike. However, they are also concerned not to look foolish in the eyes of their workmates. It is unlikely that a nurse's colleagues would discover, to the nurse's embarrassment, that they had been too cynical and untrusting of a patient. It is all too possible that those same colleagues can discover that the nurse has been too naïve, gullible and trusting. Such a public discovery can be highly embarrassing to the nurse, and effect both public reputation in the hospital, and even perhaps the view taken by managers and prospects for promotion. The safest course is, therefore, always to mistrust anything PD patients do or say. To do anything else involves not just a personal risk, but also a very public one. The promotion of negative attitudes is therefore in some sense structured into the social fabric of the High Security Hospital.

Negative attitude nurses were very much more likely to report negative impacts of work on their lives outside of hospital. A number described how they had started to view others in PD terms. These nurses reported a change in the way they viewed other people, particularly non-patients, both within and outside work. They found themselves looking for ulterior manipulative motives in others so habitually that it came to dominate their perspective of others. *They make you lose your faith in human nature a little bit at times. But, they can tend to adversely colour your opinion of people. You tend to maybe get a little over-suspicious, you tend to think, maybe think the worse, doubt people's motives, try and second-guess them, and it can be, you can become a little suspicious maybe.* Awareness of this process differed between nurses, with some referring to it as becoming cynical or even paranoid. Others related how this perspective contaminated relationships with their friends or marital partners, and how they deliberately inhibited it when they noticed themselves acting in this way, or were confronted by others with the fact they were doing so. *Sometimes people pick up on that and you get classic comments from friends and family like – 'You are not at work now, stop analysing everything I say' – which you don't realize you are doing. You have got to be careful you don't have the element of – What do they mean by that? Always second guessing people. You lose the ability to trust and take things at face value.* The suspicion can become generalized to the degree that even strangers met in the street, or people in the pub, are suspected of harbouring hidden and nasty motivations. *If you meet someone in the street, just passing, and you are just talking to them, some fellow walking his dog or whatever, and whereas before you've come here you'd walk past and 'wasn't he a nice fellow and all that'. But once you have worked here for five years – you walk by and think, 'well wasn't he a nice fellow – yeah, but.*

He might be doing this or doing that or he might just be putting a front on to be nice to us'. Nurses can become 'wary of everybody', and start to perceive PD behaviour in everyday life, judging others to be PD but remaining on the 'socially acceptable side'. It seems feasible that this suspicion may also contribute to nurses' conflict and lack of cohesion with their managers, if the managers themselves were interpreted as behaving in a deceitful and manipulative way. A few nurses suggested that constant contact with manipulative patients had rubbed off on them to the extent that they became more devious themselves, both inside and outside work. *It can make you a little bit devious, . . . you do negotiate and you do coax and compromise, you sometimes find it kind of goes over into the rest of your life as well . . . You sometimes try to manipulate situations, I think . . . You become a bit of a PD yourself.*

The comments of many nurses evidenced an increased concern for their own personal safety, with one describing how he had fists clenched with keys in between his fingers when walking up an alleyway near his local public house, in case somebody jumped out at him. Others described how they had increased home security, become more careful about locking doors or had fitted security devices. These nurses also reported being extremely wary and suspicious of people they did not know, even people on the street or in shopping centres distributing leaflets are carefully avoided. The level of tension and fear that nurses can live with is plentifully evidenced in their reported behaviour: pubs are vacated when a rough-looking customer enters; brushing shoulders with someone in a crowded street is viewed as a potential trigger of violence; and a sudden movement behind his back caused a nurse to 'jump' out of his skin (referred to colloquially by one nurse as the 'Ashworth twitch').

In a similar way to the heightened awareness of personal safety, fear for children is increased. Nurses reported that they became 'over-protective' or 'went over the top' in ensuring the safety of their children from predatory paedophiles. Children were not allowed to go out as much, or at all, unaccompanied, and any adult who sought a child's company was under immediate suspicion: *Like with me kids, somebody says 'well I'll come,' well, – why are they coming over? Why are they saying hello? Why are they coming to my kids, there's other kids around? And like my, my, my little'ns got blonde hair, which they are, they are beautiful but, you think well they're the targets, you read most notes first time it's blue-eyed, blonde-haired kids.* It is almost as if a constant consciousness of the reality of the threat to the child posed by paedophiles makes the nurses feel that they have lost their innocence, and that their view of everyday activities has been contaminated and spoiled: [It] *makes you look at things differently, family holidays like we went to* [name of place deleted]*, everybody let their kids do this and that, me as well because I have too but part of me would like to lock them in the house and never let them go out permanently because of the insight of the things that go on, am thinking sometimes that if only that mum knew, simple things like getting your kids from the pool and drying them on the side. That is fun and* *you should be able to do that but having seen and read the fantasies people have got, you keep on thinking that if only that mum knew what she was doing, that kind of thing.* Other nurses reported a more general loss of innocence not specifically related to children. Face-to-face contact with the reality of PD patients who have committed dreadful crimes made these nurses recognize that horrible things could happen in life, whether that be extreme childhood abuse or extreme offences. They were astounded that people could carry out such horrible actions, and characterized their previous selves as naïve and unknowing. At a simpler level they were made aware of 'what a lot of bad people there are in the world'.

Other interviewees reported coming home stressed. For them this meant that it took time to wind down, that when they first got home they were relatively uncommunicative and found it difficult to relax or switch off, responding to sudden loud noises with a jump. Some related how this had a deleterious impact on marital relationships. This type of stress seemed to be associated with violent incidents on the ward, verbal abuse, confrontations, self-mutilation by patients, official and unofficial complaints, and public inquiries. No nurses reported this as a continuous experience, but rather that there were times, or periods of time during their working life, when the stress had been particularly acute. In addition, others spoke of increased alcohol consumption, insomnia, nightmares, and smoking. Nurses also reported that, on occasion, they might dread coming into work because of the challenges involved in caring for PD patients.

Positive nursing in a positive organization

Positive nurses do not consider PD patients to be evil or monstrous, regardless of the nature of their index offences or the way in which they were committed. This, together with the manner that positive nurses use to deal with reading the case notes (e.g. concentrating on the person as they are now) means that positive nurses will interact more, and more normally, with PD patients. These nurses had the same emotional responses to the index offences of patients. They felt anger, fear, distaste, revulsion, disgust, etc. However. they had ways of managing these feelings, and ways to legitimize their suppression to themselves, so as not to interfere with their interaction with patients. Not only did this mean that they were better able to talk with patients, it also probably meant that they were more likely to stay in the service, rather than seek a move to a non-PD work area, or an alternative psychiatric hospital.

There is no evidence in the interviews that these nurses were less aware of what PD patients were capable of, or minimized in any way what patients had done. They had just as much to say and describe about the manipulative behaviour of PD patients, and were just as conscious of the difficult behaviours they were capable of. They were just as likely to have been seriously threatened or attacked by a PD patient at some time in their career, and commented equally with the negative nurses on the violent tendencies of the PD patients in their care. Nevertheless, for the positive nurses this did not lead to an ongoing feeling of vulnerability, perhaps because they had greater confidence in their own skills.

Indeed, they were able to explain how to handle themselves and patients during challenging confrontations. They were able to contain their own natural responses to threats, complaints or verbal abuse, and not lose their tempers and shout back. Instead they were able to turn such conflicts into therapeutic encounters. Even if they failed in so doing, and a violent incident resulted, the angry and fearful responses of positive nurses were more short term and did not lead to a permanent, embedded, cautious approach to nursing. Similarly, the acute disappointments and 'let downs' generated by patients did not, for the positive nurses, result in catastrophic disappointment and an ensuing rejection of patients and the work. On the contrary such setbacks were expected, processed, and became part of the ongoing therapeutic work.

In any case, because of their more non-judgemental, respectful attitude towards patients, it would seem likely that they elicit less abuse and violence from patients. Thus it would appear that just as negative attitudes elicit negative events, in a feedback loop, so do positive attitudes elicit positive events. Both may therefore possess the properties of self-fulfilling prophecies.

Those who saw themselves in a parental role towards PD patients provided further evidence on how positive nurses interact, with love, trust, authority, and as role models. Authority will be dealt with under a consideration of structure, showing that positive nurses enacted their authority in a different way. The love and care of the positive nurses towards PD patients was probably enhanced and supported by their moral commitments (for example, to 'universal humanity') and nursing ideology (e.g. 'individualized care'). How this translated into actual action towards patients is not clear from the interviews, but it seems likely that these nurses would spend more time in direct interaction (and express pleasure in so doing), be more tolerant of poor behaviour and struggle harder to reach an understanding of it.

With respect to trust, staff were able to describe how this could be developed. Spending time with patients in friendly chat helped to build trust: *It's, it's, I think just like by talking to them I think 'cos you know you get, are getting to know them you start by talking to them, or you make an effort to chat to or to see them on the gallery you know, and, and that walking past you or towards you or whatever, make an effort to stop and talk; say you're there, you know, if they need you and let them know that you're there, basically.* It is important to the development of trust that such contact takes place over a long period of time, and that it is carried out in such a way as to demonstrate that the nurse considers the patient to be a social equal, and does not pass judgement in any way, i.e. 'non-judgemental' and 'on the same level'. A number of nurses made the point that it is important to be reliable and dependable, delivering on even the smallest promise.

Such is the sensitivity of PD patients to rejection that forgetting the slightest thing could lead to their taking offence. Hence, to build trust, nurses needed to consistently do everything they said they were going to do, never going 'back on their word'.

Accepting and tolerating criticism from patients was also necessary to build trust. It reinforced mutual respect and demonstrated that nurses were willing to look into their own faults as well as those of patients. One nurse remarked this was personally difficult, and observed it to be also difficult for others. Nevertheless, positive nurses were more likely to see the benefits of criticism and complaints, and facilitate them, thus building greater trust. Other nurses put this in terms of being honest and being able to admit mistakes (e.g. 'I think you have to be prepared to admit when you make a mistake. Because it's, it's impossible for somebody to begin to trust you, especially someone who may be severely damaged'). Indeed, being open and honest about the reasons for a nurse's actions was seen as a key to nurturing trust. Expressing respect by negotiating on treatment plans and ward rules was also said to enhance and build trusting relationships, and this finding is elaborated further in the section following on 'structure'. Some nurses made the point that one cannot expect to be trusted if you do not give some trust. These comments were made by nurses mainly in response to being questioned on whether patients should be given responsibilities. It is clear from the context of these answers that what nurses had in mind was entrusting patients on minor matters in relation to ward tasks.

The common denominator of these methods of trust building seems to be a non-judgemental approach. If patients are not judged for their index offence or other behaviour, then the nurses will be willing to spend time with them, treat them as equals, be attentive to keeping promises, accept criticism, give honesty, negotiate treatment, and offer a little trust. All these elements of relating to patients are based upon a fundamental attitude of acceptance. Nurses found it personally rewarding when they felt they had won the trust of a PD patient. This was regarded as a difficult achievement that was not generally possible with all patients. However, when it did occur, the nurses felt good about it. The key indicator that trust had been established was that patients would approach the staff to talk about intimate matters, or more specifically their feelings. The nature of the reward for nurses in this is not fully clear, but one nurse's statement hints that it is about knowing that they have made interpersonal contact with the PD patient as a person, or that they have evoked some commitment to the social contract between people: *I think just by someone, the fact that someone wanting to, your time your experience, it is quite rewarding 'cos like oh, it means that there must be something, some element of trust, some element of, something there.* Having this trust makes daily management of the ward a much easier state of affairs, because patients will confide and share their disturbed thoughts and feelings, instead of expressing them in disruptive behaviour. Forewarning the nurses of their feelings gives the nurses an opportunity to work out alternative solutions, thus preventing harmful acts towards themselves or others.

Giving trust to patients in order to develop trust can be a risky venture. It can lay the nurses open to being manipulated or otherwise taken advantage of. Thus even those nurses who recognized that giving trust was an essential step in relationship building, recognized that it had to be realistic, small scale, cautious, and 'guarded'. However, positive nurses were significantly more willing to do this than negative nurses, who frequently operated from a position of no trust whatsoever on any occasion. The kinds of responsibilities involved were not large. The considerable number of examples given by the interviewees indicates their constrained nature, and included (depending on the ward concerned) such things as:

- deciding democratically what channel to watch on the ward TV
- being responsible for the use of their own milk supply
- taking a temporary leadership role in a therapeutic group
- having their own room key
- involvement in the Patients' Council
- organizing social activities in the Recreation Hall
- ward cleaning and tidying
- garden projects
- self-medication (inhalers) for asthma
- feeding the fish in the ward aquarium
- making their own cups of tea
- keeping their own room tidy
- attending to their own personal hygiene
- getting up in the morning and going to daily activities
- washing their own clothes.

However, although these responsibilities seem small, patients could exploit them to their personal advantage. The nurses told how patients who were given the responsibility of serving meals gave larger portions to their friends; how a patient who was given responsibility for his phone calls contacted the national press with a false story; how a patient tried to use his position on the Patients' Council to pursue a personal agenda; how a patient responsible for cleaning the kitchen refused access to patients who were messy, etc. Once again, the events reported by the Fallon Inquiry (Fallon *et al.* 1999) were given as an example by several interviewees of the risks involved in giving patients any responsibility.

Along with expressions of caution and mention of risks, nurses were also able to identify specific benefits in extending a degree of responsibility or leadership. Giving patients some responsibility was perceived as a treatment in its own right. Some saw this mainly in terms of self care – unless patients took care of their own rooms, personal hygiene, finances, etc., how could they be expected to do so on release? Most saw it in terms of giving the opportunity to change social behaviour, to exercise self control, or take into account the needs of other patients. *We had a patient here who worked in the patients' kitchen. . . . He had to be diplomatic, and also he was then caught between the staff and the other group of patients who were coming up for their food. And he would have to learn to deal with both sides of that. . . . And he now tends to feel he has a certain responsibility to the community as a whole, so that's an area that's worked for him.* The perception that giving a measured and monitored amount of responsibility to patients is therapeutic was weakly associated with an overall positive attitude to PD. Other benefits of giving patients some responsibility were identified as (a) serving an assessment function, through making visible therapeutic progress, and (b) increasing confidence and self-esteem.

Just as negative attitude nurses took away damaging personal consequences and effects from their work, positive nurses could also take away gains in personal development and psychological well-being. Nurses felt a rewarding sense of accomplishment and achievement when they were able to see patients improving, making progress in their ability to interact positively, forming relationships with staff, and moving towards discharge. *I get a kick out of it, I really do get a kick out if, I, I feel like I'm doing something, I'm achieving something, not everyday, achieving something, and they can rely on me. And if it's a day of trust then it's a day of trust. It's worth it, and I'm learning.* Or as another nurse put it, 'I'm doing a job that is having an impact upon other people's lives' as compared to his previous job which had been a 'treadmill'. Others mentioned gains in self-awareness, and related these to their work situation, describing how they had acquired a greater consciousness of the effect of their behaviour on patients and others. This was expressed in various ways, for example, 'question myself more', 'look more at myself', being less willing to 'jump to conclusions', or 'think more about the consequence of my actions'. For some this meant a process of periodically standing back and taking stock, thinking about and analysing interactions. This was about giving consideration to two areas: how the patients made them feel; and the impact that had. Both were felt to require an unusual degree of self-honesty, and awareness of how they might appear to others. The fact that some nurses are caused to reconsider themselves seems likely to be a consequence of some characteristic PD behaviour. Fairly typically, PD patients will consider themselves to be unjustly or badly treated, and will verbally challenge the nurses in a hostile, aggressive fashion. Nurses can then choose to regard this as bullying manipulation targeted at pressurizing them into relaxing ward rules, or they can examine how they themselves may have contributed, albeit unwittingly, to the confrontation. The latter course may lead to insights about the distortions of the PD perception of the world, or to a greater understanding of their own motivations.

Yet other nurses felt that working with PD patients had made them stronger in character, confidence and assertiveness. They felt that their experience had given them the ability to be more consistent, and less likely to crumble in the face of verbal pressure (e.g. 'I can sort of stand up for myself and say that's wrong and I think that's what these people have given me, the ability to face people'). As with self-awareness, this seems to be a response to dealing with the confrontations that are a perennial part of everyday interactions with PD patients. Many nurses explained their growth in strength in terms of the acquisition of skills that they did not previously have, through a process of trial and error, learning from their previous mistakes. Most referred to this growth in personal strength being displayed within the work setting only, but one interviewee reported that it had extended to being able to deal with difficult situations outside of work, while another was puzzled by the apparent paradox that he had developed this strength in the work setting, but had not otherwise changed. A similar number of nurses felt that they had gained in 'understanding', 'empathy', 'care' and 'compassion'. These feelings for PD patients hinged on two things. For some nurses the most salient was the current state of the patients – their feelings of helplessness and self-denigration, their rejection by society and judgement by others, and also their good qualities that find expression in daily life on the ward. For other nurses it was the severe childhood abuse suffered in the past by patients that evoked compassion (e.g. 'I often feel that I want to sort of just take them back to their childhood and just change everything for them. And I often wonder if that was the case how different things would be for them. But I can't do that, so . . .'). These deep musings can lead to the development of profound philosophical positions on the human condition: *We have seen a lot of the failings of the human animal here, the human race. We are not infallible – we can all be. We are very fragile and they in turn are very fragile for whatever they have done.*

Smaller numbers of nurses reported a growth of interest in PD patients, and of tolerance and patience. Those who talked about becoming interested had become intrigued by PD patient behaviour, finding a sense of fascination and a challenge to rise to the demands of caring for them. The source of greater tolerance was the same. Having to deal with difficult PD behaviour taught nurses a more patient attitude to others, that had an effect on their dealings with people outside the hospital. Reporting positive impacts from working with PD patients was very highly associated with an overall positive attitude to PD.

Structure: rules and routine

Rules and routine were referred to almost interchangeably, for many of the rules were about what could be done at what time: for example, 'lights out' times; times at which snacks, meals or drinks were available; times of access to various rooms and items; getting up in the morning and going off to activities. Other rules stipulated what items patients could not possess: for example, restrictions on the total quantity of property patients could have in their rooms; no cutlery, knives, or other potential or actual weapons; no items that could be used to harm themselves or set fires; the management and supervision of personal finances. Yet other rules were about personal conduct: for example, safety (no smoking in bedrooms); fairness (equal shares of patient resources, such as hot drinks, milk, time on the telephone); mutual respect (no violence or verbal abuse, no music late at night, smoking restricted to smoking areas); self-care (bathing, shaving and changing clothes regularly, keeping room clean and tidy). Nurses mentioned so many rules that they cannot all be quoted. Some of these rules were set centrally for the hospital as a whole, especially those related to major issues of safety and security. Other rules were set by nurses at ward level, or were specific to the function of an individual ward (e.g. admission wards were more structured than rehabilitation or parole wards). Sometimes rules had to be created on the spot as patients found new things to request or new means to challenge existing regulations. All these factors, which contribute to the controls placed on patients, are represented graphically in the 'triangle of structure' shown in Figure 6.1.

Nurses saw conformity to the rules as a problematic area. PD patients were intrinsically anti-authority, and this was remarked upon by a number of nurses (21 per cent); they were perceived to be prone to be difficult, argue back, or refuse to accept external constraints on their behaviour. 'Your typical psychopath', said one nurse, 'doesn't like rules, and doesn't like to be reminded of them either.' What is more, the nurses, because they enforce

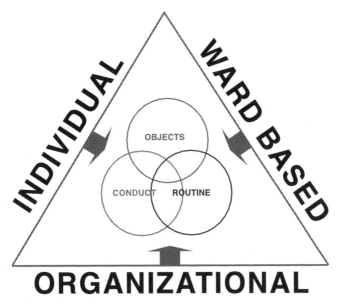

Figure 6.1 The triangle of structure.

the rules, come to be identified by PD patients as representatives of a system that has condemned them and locked them away. As a result, interactions can be very tense, and red-hot with hostility when rules are upheld. *Now property in this place is quite valuable, because it's all they have, and you step in the middle of it. Their whole anger, frustrations, everything that is, come about from, you know, society that had brought them here, and authority and everything. You're it at that particular time.* The nurses' accounts of typical PD behaviour are littered with terms such as 'rebellious', 'refuse to conform', 'disruptive', 'challenging', 'uncooperative', 'confrontational', etc.

The anti-authoritarianism of PD patients originated in childhood, according to some nurses. In particular, they expressed the view that, as children, PD patients had not been subjected to any consistent structure (rules or routine), but had instead been completely uncontrolled and undisciplined. *They have to have a, how can I put it, a regime, not a strict regime, but they need some sort of regime. Because I think that's what they've been lacking in their early years, which has obviously contributed to the situation that they're in.*

There are multiplicities of means by which patients try to challenge or subvert the control system of the hospital. Most of the strategies detailed in the section on manipulation (see p. 43) were also described by nurses as ways in which PD patients sought to undermine or break the rules: bullying, corrupting, conditioning, capitalizing, conning and dividing.

Safety and security were the primary goals and reasons for the structure imposed by nurses, with a significant number mentioning this. Security rules involved staff deployment and access restrictions to areas of the ward; fire safety, rules about cooking and smoking; room and personal searches to deter the possession of banned items; counting tools and cutlery to prevent the construction of weapons. These rules were so ubiquitous, so much part of the background expectancies of life in High Secure settings, that nurses seldom mentioned, as one of the rules, the fact that doors were locked and patients were not allowed to leave. Everybody knew this, therefore it was redundant to mention it, even in an interview with a stranger. There was no relationship between the mention of security as a rationale for structure, and overall attitudes to PD. All nurses, whatever their attitude, realized that the maintenance of security was an integral part of their role.

Apart from the obvious prevention of security breaches, effective structure was thought to have two other, more oblique impacts upon general safety: containing the informal hierarchy among patients, and minimizing the level of disruption on the wards. Effective structure, especially the imposition of equity, fairness and arbitration in between–patient disputes, was seen as preventing the exploitation of patients by each other. A full account of how patients seek to exploit each other, and construct and informal hierarchy or 'pecking order', has been provided previously. The practice is ubiquitous and appears to emerge on any ward where there are PD patients, who will bully, victimize and exploit each other unless the nurses identify it and intervene to prevent it. One interviewee described how in the past some wards had let a few patients have responsibility for food distribution (meals, tea, coffee, ward food supplies, etc.). He then reported how, on those wards, the patients in charge had given food and supplies preferentially to their friends ('those one or two patients who have served the meals, all their mates got the good, the best, cups and food and two chickens and someone else got none; some patients never saw a tea bag; and patients didn't know that biscuits came up at tea time'). When the staff finally realized it, they discovered that some patients' rooms contained vast stocks of sugar and tea for their own use, whereas other people had none!

Wards with an effective structure were also much more harmonious places in which to work, with less disruption. A 'relaxed atmosphere' was created, with everyone knowing what they were doing and when. Because the limitations on conduct and possessions were understood, there was less friction between staff and patients, and between the patients themselves. Thus everything was calmer, quieter and 'the ward runs like clockwork'. As a result, nurses themselves felt more secure, and patients had a platform from which they found it easier to engage in the treatment that was offered. Moreover, because there was less disruption, not only the stress but also the workload of nurses was reduced, with fewer crises and less friction to be actively managed.

Structure as therapy

This link between effective structure and therapy emerged during the interviews in different respects. There were five ways in which nurses considered that structure made an impact upon the treatment of PD patients. This was either directly, through a psychological effect upon the disorder itself, or via enhancement of patient confidence in staff, general stability, and therapeutic engagement.

Predictability

The predictability and certainty of a structured environment was seen as producing a feeling of security in PD patients, who were perceived as disliking change and being much more comfortable with stability. Patients were seen as wanting, even at times requesting, a highly structured environment, with clear, consistent, and stable rules and routines. The opposite, an environment where, for whatever reason, the patients did not know what the consequences of actions were, or what would happen next, was considered to be highly stressful for people with a PD.

Cognitive clarity

These nurses viewed PD patients as psychologically chaotic and out of control. External controls provided by the structure of rules and daily activity were considered to imbue internal psychological control and calm orderliness. *A lot of these patients . . . their previous experiences have been chaotic. And in order for them to deal with their own internal chaos they need an external structure where they can feel safe.* Without that external structure in place to hold them together, PD patients may 'break down', become disruptive and disorderly, or get 'carried away'. One nurse explicitly described using this as a treatment method: *With the majority of PD patients, there is an element of chaos there, in their behaviours and emotions, away from chaotic backgrounds. Talking to many PDs, they create this confusion, complaints; litigation; allegations; inappropriate behaviours. I mean they are responsible for their actions but they feel they have no control over it and it's almost subconscious actions that they are doing. To give them structure is almost like taking some of the responsibility for the behaviours off them. Initially, that is very important because you can deal with things in piecemeal then and you can break issues down.*

Relationship clarity

This meant that patients had to know and understand the limitations of the relationships that they could have with nurses. That knowledge and understanding would avoid any confusion and misapprehension, and prevent the development of conditioning relationships.

Feeling safe

An effective structure was perceived by these nurses as producing a sense of safety in PD patients. This was two-fold. Patients were confident that whatever they did, the nurses could contain the situation in a safe manner without anyone being hurt. Secondly, they were secure in the knowledge that the staff would deal with any other patients who were threatening, aggressive or exploitative. *A lot of personality disorder patients often don't feel safe either from other patients. . . . Sometimes they don't feel safe about what they might do. You know if there isn't somebody who can deal with those situations when they arise, then it would be left to . . . it's like a bad situation.*

Sense of purpose

These nurses argued that a sense of purpose could be externally provided and led by the staff through a structured regime of care, and that the PD patients specifically responded to this with better self-care, greater self-respect and increased engagement in therapeutic activities. *I think you have to give a bit of push, and if you, if you've got a bit of an organized regime, they'll follow it. And that you'll find you'll get a better response, you'll see them coming out better.*

There was no relationship between drawing this link between structure and treatment, and overall attitude to PD. This was an unexpected finding, as it was considered that holding this point of view would increase the nurses' sense of purpose in doing their work. Alternatively, it may have made sense for this idea to correlate with a negative attitude, as it places an intrinsic value on authority and hierarchy. Neither was the case, and this may be because the link between structure and therapy was seldom fully articulated. In many cases it was implicit rather than explicit in the way nurses described their work in keeping order.

In addition to these five ways in which some nurses considered structure had a direct therapeutic impact, a number of nurses also viewed the internal structure of the hospital as rehabilitative. This view was also not related to overall attitude to PD. Structure (rules and routine) are seen by these nurses both as a reflection of the way things are in the 'real world' outside the hospital, and as a means by which PD patients can be rehabilitated in a behavioural sense. By training them to adhere to a regular routine, and abide by rules, nurses see themselves as preparing patients for discharge. Ability to comply with the structure inside the hospital is seen as a demonstration of capability to comply with social norms outside. Thus, each time a nurse imposed a rule or required compliance, this could be viewed not only as keeping order within the hospital, but also as a therapeutic learning experience. *Gives them the opportunity to learn to live within a set of rules, which they would have to if they were outside. Community – the outside community, society – has a set of rules which you and I have to live up to and they would have to conform to. So, in here, having a structure like that gives them the opportunity to put it in practice, to learn.*

Putting these ideas together results in the speculative model (Figure 6.2) of the relationship between structure and therapy for PD patients. Thus, in the view of the interviewed nurses, there was a four-fold impact of structure on therapeutic progress with PD patients. Firstly, it produced stability on the ward, a prerequisite for any therapeutic work whatsoever. Secondly, it provided a rehabilitative framework through which patients could be exposed to increasingly difficult tasks mirroring life in the real world. Thirdly, it increased the confidence of patients in the staff, enhancing their willingness to engage with treatment. Fourthly, structure was perceived to have a direct therapeutic impact in its own right.

It must be stressed that the question of whether structure does have a therapeutic impact of its own on PD has not been answered by this research. Figure 6.2 has been extracted and combined from the related ideas of the many nurses who consider that it does. Whether this is the case remains an open question.

A significant number of the nurses interviewed indicated that too much structure could, in itself, be anti-therapeutic. An over-organized ward presents few opportunities for choice, reduces interaction because everything

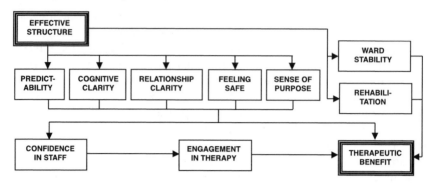

Figure 6.2 Model of structure/therapy relationships.

is predictable, increases dependency on the hospital environment and creates institutionalism. Some nurses went on to argue that an overly prescriptive and stable environment could increase the psychological fragility of PD patients in the face of change. Too much structure would mean that the ward failed to reflect accurately a reality of social life outside of hospital, which consists of a mixture of choice and constraint. *If they accept that nurses organize the ward, run the ward, it certainly makes the ward run more smoothly. Conversely to that, I don't necessarily think that it is a good thing that nursing staff organize everything for the patients and rule every aspect of their day, because that leads to extremely institutionalized people five or ten years down the line.*

Achieving effective structure

Two means by which nurses worked to achieve an effective structure can be discerned in the interviews: practical and ethical. The practical way is by reducing uncertainty through clarity (no ambiguity, consistency between staff, infrequent change, and assertion). The ethical way is by attaining legitimacy for the structure in the eyes of patients through high standards of staff conduct (equality, honesty and integrity, equity, and bravery). These are not entirely separable, and overlap to some degree, as will be seen. Distinguishing the two in this way is purely a device for making them easier to explain, and does not imply that effective structure can be attained by either alone.

The practical route

Structure needs to be absolutely clear, without ambiguity, to all parties concerned, both staff and patients. *Because, one thing you do need is clear parameters, clear boundaries, so you know and they know that these are the rules we work within.... I think it's important to have ground rules and to have, yeah, some kind of structure that you can work within that is clearly defined to both you and the patient.* Not only did the rules themselves need to be clear, but also the consequences for the patient if they broke them. If the structure was unclear, staff would be reluctant to confront patients, and inconsistencies between staff would appear. In addition, the nurses reported that in these circumstances patients would bring pressure to bear and seek to exploit any grey areas in the rules. *Ward rules have got to be very clear. If there's any grey areas then they'll exploit that, and then you're not so sure, or can they, can't they? And it puts you on the back foot, whereas if the ward rules are very clear then it's either yes or no and it saves a hell of a lot of trouble.* The same nurse went on to point out that disputes over the rules could cause arguments and might even escalate into serious incidents of violence or disorder.

In addition all staff needed to implement the same rules in the same way, all the time. This also meant that when a nurse challenged a patient on a failure to adhere to a rule or policy, the active backing of the rest of the nursing team would be received. Without this consistency, patients could seek out 'weak links', or divide the staff team into two camps that disputed with each other, leaving the patients free to do what they wanted. At the very least, any inconsistency gave patients an argument that could be used to pressure staff to relax regulations. More serious problems could arise when the nurse in charge did not support the rest of the team, or when there was inconsistency between shifts, or between nurses and other disciplines, or between the ward nurses and their managers. These types of inconsistency have been previously described, together with the depression of morale that follows. Just as with lack of clarity, nurses pointed out that inconsistencies between staff lead to arguments, and arguments could lead to serious conflict or to erosion of the rules. *You need to have guidelines and boundaries that everybody sticks to, you know continuity that's what you need. You need continuity through, through all the nurses here. So, you know, if you're going to say something, you know, that the rest of the team are going to do that rather than a patient coming up and saying 'Well hang on, you're saying this but yesterday it was different, I could do this, that and the other, and you're saying "No", so you must be the bad guy', so, you know, you need good continuity.* Mention by nurses of the need for a consistent approach correlated highly with an overall positive attitude to PD, indicating that such nurses were probably better able to manage and contain patients within an effective structure.

Some nurses indicated that a stable structure, without frequent changes, was helpful and more likely to be respected by patients. *A lot of them like to know where they stand. I think that certainly one of the problems with the hospital now is a lot of the time patients don't actually know where they stand on something, and unfortunately the staff can't tell them 'cos it changes from day to day, within this hospital. Sometimes the staff don't know where they stand never mind where the patients stand.* However many more of the interviewees talked about a need to assert the rules by confronting patients and exerting pressure in order to promote conformity with the regime. The willingness to confront is similar to the ethic of bravery detailed more fully as part of the ethical route to effective structure. Examples of means to exert control over patients given by the interviewed nurses were as follows:

Reminding the patient of the rules   But you have to point it out to them, 'you're not allowed to do that', 'oh sorry, I forgot'.

Reprimanding the patient, or telling them off   They know they can or cannot do such and such a thing and they are doing it and shouldn't be doing it. They know they are going to be told off or whatever.

Seclusion   He was obviously placed in seclusion, because he was threatening, and he was being very abusive, and physically threatening, and given the opportunity he would have assaulted a member of staff.

Loss of ground parole   A lot of them will break the, in my own experience, broke the rules . . . , it would be removal of parole card status.

Prevention of social activity   You'll say to them, if, like if they don't go to their work places you know, we'll stop their social gatherings.

Loss of room key   On here they have their own room access, they're allowed their own room key, . . . There's certain conditions that they've got to sort of abide by if you like, otherwise they lose that privilege.

Reduction on stages system   A method of regulation based upon varying a patient's ability to earn wages. And then, for good behaviour and that the stages go up and obviously the more stages they get, the higher their pay is.

Calm discussion, away from others   Well I was able to talk to the patient in question and get him to realize that his behaviour was unreasonable and, and, and would not be accepted and he saw the sense in it.

Temporary removal of desirable property   e.g. tobacco, lighter, video. If you smash up that dining room, you're going to lose your TV for two days.

Ward grading system   Some wards are more structured, more restrictive than others, and persistent poor behaviour can lead to transfer to a more structured ward, the system forming a therapeutic ladder as well as a means of matching the patient to the right therapeutic environment.

Use of peer pressure *If a patient down the corridor starts playing loud music now when the ward policy agreed that all music should stop at 9 o'clock, this patient will face peer pressure from other patients alone and the staff can support that.*

Infraction of rules recorded in patient's notes Potentially affecting that person's assessment for discharge. *If a patient's behaviour is inappropriate, . . . it's just written down in the notes.*

If these control methods are split into verbal means, or those that can be considered in the broadest sense as sanctions, then mention of the latter was weakly associated with a negative overall attitude to PD. This is in agreement with the analysis of violent incidents in hospital, where a similar relationship was found between the recommendation of sanctions as a method of control and overall negative attitude.

The ethical route

The word equality brings together four ways in which nurses demonstrated to patients that they were valued, respected, and equal human beings, even though the nurses were in a position of authority and the patients had committed serious crimes. This equality was demonstrated in the way in which structure was accomplished.

Explanation The reasons behind rules and routines were fully explained to patients. *You've offered a full explanation to your patients and explained why and you can't do any more than that . . . And I, I, I just think that you've got to, you've just got to do the decent thing you've just got to be decent. . . . Well they feel valued don't they? If you, it's just valuing people as, as I would you, why would I be any different to a member of staff than a patient? Why should a staff have a full explanation and not a patient?*

Patient voice The patients' opinions and feedback about the rules were heard, listened to, and where possible there was a response. This could mean simply providing time and space for patients to express themselves, but could extend to their voting democratically (e.g. which TV channel to watch, or what time hot drinks will be served), or proposing changes to the ward rules which were then enacted (e.g. changes to the ward smoking areas).

Admission of fallibility Willingness to admit that nurses are fallible and make mistakes sometimes. There were bad judgement calls about the interpretation of rules, or the team was sometimes inconsistent about an issue, etc. *I think you have to be prepared to admit when you make a mistake. Because it's, it's impossible for somebody to begin to trust you, especially someone who may be severely damaged, if you're already playing the power game by saying they can be wrong but you can't.*

Appeal reminder   Patients were made aware that they have rights to appeal against the structure if they so wished, and nurses informed them how to do this via formal or informal complaints, the advocacy service, or the Patients' Council, etc. *I think that's important if you're going to have any smooth running. They have to have confidence in the staff, and feel that they're being treated fairly . . . a knowledge of the way which they can take a problem forward, and that might be the community meeting, or the complaints department. And, and to demonstrate that they receive fair and just outcomes.*

Nurses made considerable reference to the opposite attitude leading to serious conflicts and problems. These would occur when nurses were authoritarian, hierarchical, gave no explanation, engaged in no negotiation, considered themselves to be infallible, and issued commands 'like policemen'. Expression of equal status *vis-à-vis* PD patients is very strongly associated with overall positive attitude.

The responses that mentioned honesty and integrity covered a number of related areas. It could mean telling the patient the true reason for a rule or course of action, and in this sense it could also mean being willing to confront patients with the way their behaviour was perceived by others. More particularly it meant being constant, consistent over time: *If you say something one day and come back the next day and say something different, they remember it and they are angry.* Or it could mean the absence of any gap between rhetoric and reality, delivering on the nursing role: *Where as if it's like, if staff are consistent in what they say and what they do and how they deal with something, that's what a person needs rather than regimented things.* Nurses referred to this as 'basic genuineness', being 'direct', refusing to hide behind technical psychiatric 'jargon', not concealing their emotional reactions to patient behaviour. In other senses, honesty and integrity meant not giving false excuses for not doing things for patients, or it meant delivering on promises and commitments. Arguing for the importance of honesty and integrity in the achievement of effective structure was very highly associated with overall positive attitude to PD.

Nurses who talked about equity emphasized that patients should all be treated equally, or the same. Partly this was about making sure that some patients did not exploit others, or about ensuring an even distribution of ward tasks. *So to implement a rota and each of them to take their turn at doing it, it works well, I think it works brilliant, and they don't mind.* However it was also about not singling out or treating differently any one patient or group of patients. Potential candidates for different treatment were:

- PD patients themselves, in comparison to other diagnostic groups. *But I don't single them out and think to myself oh, she's a so and so and she's a so and so or whatever.*
- Patients who had committed particularly heinous crimes. *I mean you get people who come here who have done horrendous crimes, you know, to often the weakest victims you could possibly think of. I think everybody tries to remain in some ways non-judgemental and try and treat people as fairly as possible.*
- Patients who had violently attacked nurses. *I mean you were saying about staff getting hurt, you have to come to work the next day and you have to try and put that to the back of your mind. 'Cos you could think to yourself, well I'm not having anything else to do with her 'cos she smacked so and so and what have you.*

There was no association between the mention of the need for equity and overall attitude to PD.

Other nurses spoke about the need to be brave, and stressed that it was necessary to assert themselves, to actively confront patients who were not complying with the structure. To do this, they suggested, required courage and needed to be carried out in a non-dictatorial, non-aggressive manner, which one nurse referred to as 'the art of confrontation'. *I think you've got to be quite assertive, that you've got to be quietly confident without being over the top. You've certainly got to stand your ground.* Some of the nurses making this argument indicated that to be assertive in this way was very difficult, but that it generated respect. The difficulty arose from the potentially aversive response from patients, who may shout, swear, argue, or become violent. Mention of the need for bravery in achieving effective structure was associated with an overall positive attitude to PD.

There was a common set of nursing phrases used in the interviews in relation to both the practical and ethical routes to achieving structure:

- Staff need to have 'clear boundaries'. Depending on context, this means clarity and/or consistency between staff, or the creation of cognitive or relationship clarity.
- Patients should 'know where they stand'. This also varies in meaning by context. It can mean that patients should know the rules in advance, and that they should be unambiguous. In other contexts the phrase is used to highlight the willingness of staff to confront patients (i.e. bravery), or consistent application of the structure.
- Staff should be 'firm but fair'. This can mean bravery as detailed above, or assertion. Being fair can mean any of the factors described above as the ethical route to effective structure.

In the course of discussing structure, nurses sometimes gave an opinion about whether they were satisfied with the regulation of patients in their own wards or hospitals. These responses were readily classified into two types: (a) nurses who were satisfied with what they saw as a currently highly structured environment, or asserted that more structure was required (30 per cent), and (b) nurses who were satisfied with what they saw as a currently flexibly structured environment, or asserted that more flexibility or liberalism was required (16 per cent). Highly structured in this context meant more rules and regulations, and a more rigorous routine more strictly applied. Nurses who expressed a preference for more highly structured environments were much more likely to have a negative overall attitude to PD, perhaps reflecting their feelings of vulnerability in the face of PD patients and their behaviour.

The end results of failing to structure the ward effectively were well described by nurses. They explained that if staff did not have a clear and stable structure, consistently applied, bravely and assertively imposed in a spirit of equality, honesty, integrity, and equity, then there were potentially serious consequences. In those circumstances, the ward could descend into chaos and anarchy, in which the patients ran the ward, dictated to staff, routine broke down and patients 'ran riot'. As a further consequence the ward would be continuously disrupted; manipulation, bullying and violence would increase; therapeutic activity would cease; patients would refuse to cooperate with their treatment plans; and breaches in security would occur with patients acquiring banned items. The interviewees gave a number of examples of their experience of this occurring to one degree or another, typically saying how difficult it was to regain full control once the structure had begun to be eroded. A few stressed the need for constant vigilance and alertness to make sure that the gradual slide into this sort of situation did not occur. The premier example given by staff was that of Lawrence ward at Ashworth Hospital, the subject of the then recent Fallon Inquiry: *Other-wise they* [the PD patients] *just get carried away and they lose all track of where they are and what's appropriate and what's not appropriate and before you know it you've got, all hell's let loose on the ward. That is just chaos. The staff didn't know what was happening half the time. Because the patients ran the ward. They ran the whole community themselves. Staff were basically there just to open and close doors.* There was no relationship between mentioning the consequences of ineffective structure and overall attitude to PD. Nurses of all attitudes were equally aware of the dangers and the requirement to maintain control.

Summary

It can be clearly seen that having a positive or a negative overall attitude to PD is not simply a matter of feeling better or worse at work. Those attitudes had a clear connection to the ways nurses behaved with PD patients, to the stance they took on the keeping of good order, and to the impact that their work had on themselves and their social lives outside of work.

The positive nurses not only enjoyed their work more, but felt safer when at work, were more accepting of PD patients, had a sense of purpose and felt enthusiastic. Because of those attitudes these staff interacted more with patients, both normally and therapeutically. They were probably more likely to stay in the service, rather than take opportunities to leave and move on. When faced with the difficult behaviour of PD patients, they were able to turn conflict and confrontation into therapeutic encounter, rather than lose their tempers or respond at an emotional level. Taking their responses as a whole, it seemed likely that they elicited less confrontation from patients than did negative attitude staff. When disappointed by setbacks in progress, or antagonistic behaviour from a patient to whom they had committed much energy and time, they responded with patience and renewed effort rather than retreated to cynical pessimism. They invested more time with patients, struggled harder to understand them, and were more tolerant of their difficult behaviour. Partly due to the time they spent with patients (plus their dependability, honesty, qualified willingness to give a little trust, and their acceptance of criticism), positive nurses were more successful at winning the trust of this very mistrustful group. That in itself led to a further sense of reward and enjoyment, and to enhanced communication from patients that enabled these nurses more therapeutically to contain their behaviour.

For the positive nurses, these benefits extended outside of work. They carried away a sense of reward and accomplishment from what they had been doing, and they grew in self-awareness and understanding of others. Because of the difficulties that they managed and overcame in their interaction with patients, they grew in confidence, character and assertiveness. They also reported making gains in an understanding of and compassion for others, and in patience and tolerance.

There was little support in the findings of this study for any assertion that positive attitude nurses were soft and weak, or poor at managing and controlling patients. They had just as much to say about the violent and manipulative behaviour of PD patients. They were equally as aware of the necessity to maintain safety and security, and were equally as able to describe what happened when ward structure broke down. Yet their method of achieving effective structure was differently accented from that of the negative attitude nurses. The positive nurses saw certain elements of both the practical and ethical routes as being more important than others. These were: consistency between different staff members, human equality between staff and patients, honesty and integrity in applying the rules, and courage in confronting patients.

Similarly, the negative attitude nurses did not just feel differently about their work – loathing it, feeling vulnerable, rejecting of patients, accompanied by feelings of futility and exhaustion. Because of these attitudes they interacted less with patients, deliberately avoiding them on occasion. They were more likely to hold angry feelings, considering the PD patients to be bad, evil and blameworthy. Those feelings probably leaked, either verbally or non-verbally, causing more conflict. That conflict was not so well handled, and was more likely to elicit uncontrolled negative emotions from this group of staff through, for example, loss of temper and self-control. Setbacks with patients, or their difficult behaviour, were more likely to lead to these staff being complacent, leaving the service or no longer trying to engage therapeutically with patients. For the negative nurses mistrust and cynicism were pervasive, and they were unwilling to extend even the smallest degree of controlled trust.

For the negative nurses the costs of working with PD patients were high, and the impact extended outside of the work setting. They started to view friends and kin in PD terms, continually searching for manipulative ulterior motives in their behaviour, becoming suspicious and even slightly paranoid, particularly of strangers. They became more conscious of their own and their families' vulnerability to crime, and in particular became very protective of their children. The negative attitude nurses also reported a number of additional signs of personal stress.

There is insufficient evidence to say that negative attitude nurses were worse at accomplishing effective ward structure, although this does seem possible. They were much more hostile and angry towards patients, but also more likely to avoid them, less likely to speak about the need for courageously confronting them, and definitely less likely to express the need to ethically legitimate their authority in the eyes of patients. Instead they expressed more reliance upon systems of reward and punishment – a view that could be called 'crude behaviourism' – and were more likely to prefer a more structured environment for patients.

7 Us and them

A thorough description of life and work with PD patients in the High Security Hospitals has now been provided. In the opening chapters the nature of PD, negative professional attitudes to PD patients, the organization of forensic psychiatric services for PD serious offenders, and their nursing care were all described. Through the intervening chapters, the challenges presented by PD patients to their carers have been presented, with information about how some nurses manage those challenges more positively. The roles of the hospital organization, and the clinical team, have been shown to either help or hinder positive attitudes. Furthermore, the attitudes of staff have been shown to have impacts within the ward and in the personal lives of staff.

It is now time to turn to the lessons that can be learned from the findings of this study. For the first time the factors that underlie or provide a foundation for positive attitudes to PD offenders have been described in detail. Many of these carry clear implications for services, managers and individual practitioners of every psychiatric discipline. It is also likely that there are many lessons here that may be equally applicable to the psychiatric management of PD patients in general psychiatry, both in acute psychiatric wards, and in the community. Lastly, placed in a wider context, the results of this study raise questions about the attitudes and beliefs of society as a whole, towards and about PD. For example, does our society have a positive attitude towards the sufferers of PD, and to what extent are our institutions imbued with the same moral commitments and values that distinguish the positive nurses described in this study? After the key findings of this research have been pulled together into a single model, these questions will be examined.

Model of attitude to PD

Trying to draw together the findings of this piece of research, *in toto*, is a daunting prospect. It is clearly necessary to simplify and condense the findings to examine how they may relate to each other. However that process of simplification provokes deep anxiety, as it is possible that the results are given a shape not completely justified by their extent and detail. Nevertheless, an effort must be made in this direction, at the very least to provide a picture around which further debate and research can be assembled.

With this in mind, Figure 7.1 has been devised as the best way, in my current opinion, to show how the results of this study cohere and produce a meaningful pattern. At the same time, I wish to acknowledge that the reality is likely to be much more complex than this simplified diagram implies. Causes and effects are probably much more densely interwoven. The mechanisms, psychological and social, out of which attitudes to PD grow, seem likely to be related and interacting over time. In thinking about how to display this diagrammatically, I considered portraying them as interlocking bricks in a structure supporting positive attitude, or as columns supporting the roof of a classical temple, or as the individual cells of a complete honeycomb. Perhaps the reader could bear these alternative pictures in mind while considering the model.

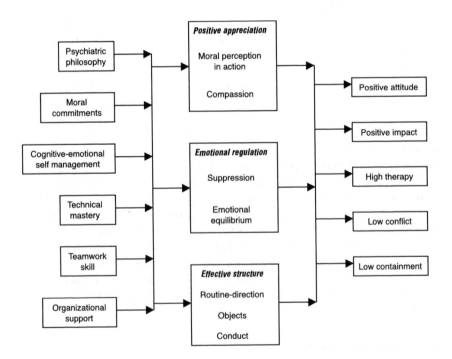

Figure 7.1 Diagrammatic results of the study. The left-hand column shows the under-lying mechanisms or foundations for positive attitudes to PD patients; the centre column shows the processes accomplished via those underlying mechanisms; and the right-hand column shows the outcomes of those processes.

Underlying mechanisms or foundations

Psychiatric philosophy

A particular set of beliefs and conceptions about psychiatry and the work of psychiatric nurses supports positive attitudes. These include belief in and commitment to the importance of psychosocial factors in the cause of PD, and in the efficacy of treatment in producing improvements in patients' behaviour. These beliefs cohere with others, giving nurses the capacity to understand the difficult behaviours of PD patients in a psychological way, rather than becoming angry and blaming them. This overall psychiatric philosophy is bedded in a focus on individuals, viewing their personal development and psychiatric problems as, in some sense, unique to them – a view which also fits with an appreciation of the role of abuse as a child in producing the type of person we call PD. This particular philosophy means that the nurses who hold it view themselves as professional agents of psychological change, and the hospital as a secure location for that psychosocial treatment, thus preventing future crime. When under pressure from patients and their behaviour, they are able to keep that view in mind.

Moral commitments

A further key foundation for positive attitudes is a set of moral choices or commitments made or acquired by the nurses. These included honesty (even when it was difficult or costly), bravery (being willing to confront patients and risk violence when necessary), equality (demonstrating through a variety of ways a lack of superiority), non-judgementalism (eschewing large-scale moral valuation of the patient), universal humanity (expression of an inclusive picture of the human race and a valuing of people despite their diversity), and individual value (an appreciation of the value of the individual person). Possibly linked to these moral positions is the way nurses identify themselves as fulfilling a parental role towards PD patients, especially in the provision of care and nurturance.

Cognitive-emotional self-management

These are a range of techniques either deployed through an inner dialogue, self-reminders, or even by habitual and ingrained ways of thinking. As such they include some of the moral and philosophical positions described above, which are consciously used by some nurses to help them to manage their emotional reactions to patients, or to correct their perception of them. However, they also include additional techniques such as concentration on the patients as they are now rather than what they had done in the past; getting to know the patients first before finding out about their index offences; drawing a distinction between the individuals and their behaviour; perseverance; and bearing in mind the expectation that patients will let the nurse down.

Technical mastery

This involves interpersonal skills that enable positive attitudes to PD, and include mastery of the art of confrontation, knowing how to stay calm and to reason with aroused patients, the ability to give neutral feedback about their behaviour, thus being able to turn conflict into therapeutic learning. A similar skill is visible in the facilitation of complaints as a therapeutic method in its own right, or in the de-escalation of imminently violent situations via verbal interaction.

Teamwork skill

The ways in which the nursing and multidisciplinary teams work together also sustain positive attitudes. Taking good feelings from the support of co-workers into the interaction with patients and, vice versa, taking away negative affect from that interaction and ventilating it with colleagues (reciprocal emotional pumping) enables a positive approach to prevail. In addition, sharing the burden of care, which can at times of ongoing difficulty be intense, is another team skill that assists everyone. Finally, the accomplishment of consistency in relation to the rules and routine for patient conduct cannot be achieved on an individual basis, but is a team skill that facilitates positive working on the part of the individual.

Organizational support

This final ingredient appears to be crucial, with the survey showing that it is a vital contributor to the overall attitude of staff to PD patients. Key elements identified by this study include policy clarity and stability around rules for patient conduct, the provision of specialist training (in professional preparation, on induction to PD care, and post-basic), an effective organization of clinical supervision for front-line clinical staff, and a management that is deeply integrated into clinical care, with a presence on the wards and explanations provided for necessary management actions.

Processes accomplished

Positive appreciation

Because of their psychological understanding, psychiatric philosophy, and moral commitments, positive attitude nurses are able to positively appreciate PD patients as valued human beings, and feel compassion for them in their disability.

Emotional regulation

Through similar means, and through technical mastery, teamwork skill and cognitive-emotional self-management, nurses are able to suppress their natural responses towards the past actions and current behaviours of PD patients, setting them to one side and maintaining their own emotional equilibrium. They are thus enabled to deal more effectively and calmly with the difficult patient management situations that confront them on a regular basis.

Effective structure

Through the whole range of actions that go to make up the foundations of a positive attitude, nurses are enabled to operate from a legitimated ethical standpoint, and create an effective structure for ward life, including a routine for patients that has direction, and rules about restrictions on objects and behaviour that are consistently applied.

Outcomes

Positive attitude

Staff enjoy their work, feel reasonably safe and secure, are accepting of PD patients, have a sense of purpose and are enthusiastic.

Positive impact

Staff are less damaged by working with PD patients; instead of taking away feelings of vulnerability and suspicion, they become more confident, stronger, grow in self-awareness, and develop a sense of accomplishment and pride in their work.

High therapy

Because of this positive valuation, and because they are able to deal with their own emotional responses, they spend more time in the company of patients, and interact more. When difficult behaviour arises, they are able to turn that difficulty into an opportunity for therapy. At the same time the effectively structured environment may have a therapeutic impact in its own right, as well as making other therapeutic approaches both possible to organize and perhaps more likely to succeed.

Low conflict

This more positive approach means that there is less conflict overall, with a contained patient hierarchy, less violence, less manipulation, and a stable ward environment. When these conflicts do occur they are skilfully converted into therapeutic encounters.

Low containment

As nurses are more engaged with patients, positively valuing them, and are more technically skilful, providing an effectively structured environment, there is less need to contain difficult behaviour through seclusion, special observation, extra medication, etc.

The mirror image

The reverse or mirror image of this model is all too easy to describe. Staff hold a philosophy of care that stresses physiological causation, and consider treatment to be ineffective. They do not have the moral commitments that enable more nurses to be positive; nor do they have the self-management methods that enable others to cope with their emotional responses to patients' actions, past and present. They are interpersonally unskilled, handicapping their efforts to interact with patients and deal with their behaviour. They work within teams that are poorly coordinated, without effective mutual support and collaboration. They are also failed by an organization that leaves them isolated in the face of PD patients, without regular clinical supervision or appropriate training, within a hierarchy where the responsibility for rules is ambiguous and unclear. In consequence these nurses are unable to value PD patients, instead rejecting and avoiding interaction with them. They are unable to regulate their own emotional responses, so that angry and judgemental feelings towards patients become deeply embedded in their overall attitude. Their work within an ineffective structure, with ambiguous rules, inconsistent staff, and an uncertain routine, leaves them isolated and unable to function. They therefore loathe their work, feel exposed and vulnerable, are rejecting of patients, pessimistic and exhausted. The work damages their own psychological functioning, deeply impacting upon the way they view themselves and others, leading to feelings of fear and vulnerability not just for themselves but also for their families. Opportunities for therapy are missed, or undermined by an ineffective ward structure. Conflict between patients, and between patients and staff, is frequent and intense, with a consequent high level of containment strategies in use (e.g. seclusion).

Implications for hospitals and DSPD services

Part of the problem with the above depiction of attitudes to PD is that it presents two polar opposites: the positive staff possessed of all the right beliefs, commitments and skills, found wanting in the negative staff. That description is fine as a didactic device, but carries dangers if it is literally interpreted. Within the highly charged environment of the High Security Hospitals in the UK, such black and white thinking can lead managers to interpret their mission as one of locating and removing the 'bad' staff – a strategy that may be divisive and create further conflict. Clearly, perceiving things in this way also means that the manipulative stance of PD patients finds fertile ground and a sympathetic hearing. However, both the questionnaire and interview surveys have demonstrated that attitude to PD was normally distributed, with few staff at either end of the continuum, and most spread across the middle. Moreover, those attitudes were found to be organizationally as well as individually determined, with much that services could do to promote more positive approaches.

One potentially striking conclusion from this study is that negative reactions to PD people are normal. They behave in very challenging ways, do obnoxious things, and as a result arouse angry and fearful feelings. This study showed that negative attitude nurses were not doing something qualitatively different, they were simply failing to do what positive nurses did. The implication is that the positive staff had, in some way, found a path that enabled them to move forward in a beneficial way with their patients, a path simply not found by the negative nurses. Their attitudes need to be overcome, but they are natural and should not lead to blame or rejection of nurses who show them. Instead what should be encouraged, and supplied, is education, supervision, challenge, development and growth.

A starting point for change would be in the basic training of the psychiatric professionals involved in the care of PD patients. Responses in the interviews indicated that training content on the nature of PD, treatment approaches, etc., was patchy, variable, and occasionally absent. In the absence of training, staff pick up attitudes and beliefs from those with whom they work. Given the predominantly negative attitude to PD embedded in all professional psychiatric disciplinary cultures, this maintains the status quo. If overall attitudes are to change, then the educational preparation of workers must improve in terms of the quantity and quality of content about PD. The requirements for the different psychiatric professions will vary, but all should be supplied with the intellectual equipment to identify PD behaviour, possess a range of alternative psychological understandings to interpret that behaviour, and have the opportunity to develop the necessary skills to deal with it within the context of their particular role. The overall philosophy of that training needs to inculcate the values that have been shown by this study to be associated with positive attitudes. It also needs to assert optimism and hope about the potential of treatment, and thoroughly explore the potential of psychosocial explanations of the disorder.

Although this is easily written, it is not likely to be easily put into practice. Take, for example, the issue of what I have called 'psychiatric philosophy'. This includes a focus upon nurture causes for PD, and a belief in treatment efficacy. Yet there is, at present, only partial evidence for the former, and little firm evidence at all for the latter. For this reason, many authorities and psychiatric professionals are prone to take up negative and pessimistic outlooks on PD psychiatric care and treatment. However, the evidential position is not supportive of this stance either. The simple fact is that we don't really know. Therefore, because of the ways in which pessimistic perspectives enhance the whole range of overall negative attitude here described, it behoves all senior teaching and research personnel to be cautious and responsible in the way in which the evidence is presented, at conferences, in their writings, and in their training of junior staff.

The problem of securing the best psychiatric philosophy is perhaps more acute for some psychiatric professions than for others. Medical psychiatry in the UK (and in many other places) has a strong affiliation to organic explanations of mental disorders. That profession also focuses upon psychiatric diagnosis as the first step in care – a move that promotes seeing people as expressions of a type, rather than as individuals in their own right. These allegiances and practices run counter to those which have been shown in this research to promote overall positive attitudes to PD. In addition, some psychiatrists reject the idea that PD is a mental disorder, or a condition that merits psychiatric treatment. As I have argued in a previous work (Bowers 1998), there is no way finally to resolve this argument: simply a decision has to be taken whether treating PD as a mental disorder has superior consequences to not doing so.

A further challenge is the inculcation of those moral values that underpin positive attitudes. This means, possibly, the renewed use of small group learning, experiential learning, personal reflection, and giving feedback or accepting it from others. A reorientation of professional education in this direction would be costly and require the partial abandonment of reliance on formal lectures to large groups. Some of this type of learning is available in the training for some disciplines, but is almost entirely absent in others. Where available, it is unsystematic, probably of variable efficiency, and has not been rigorously evaluated.

The challenge goes even further than education, for we also need to examine the culture of psychiatry and the psychiatric disciplines. How moral values are established and embedded within the culture of a profession, an organization, or a service sector like psychiatry, appears to be unknown and unstudied. Presumably those moral values that find expression within psychiatry do not come out of nowhere. There must be a professionalization process through which they are passed on from one generation to another as part of the 'hidden curriculum' of becoming a psychologist, psychiatrist, social worker, prison officer or psychiatric nurse. If we can identify how this happens, then it would open up the possibility for control, or at the least, influence, in a positive direction.

Further challenges arise out of other findings from this research. For example, the capacity to psychologically understand difficult PD behaviours has been shown to be of some importance, as is technical mastery in the interpersonal skills of its management. This has multiple implications: it implies that all disciplines dealing with PD patients require a thorough grounding in psychological models of the condition; for example, cognitive-behavioural and psychodynamic models, and all their variants. Instruction needs to be deeply and firmly embedded so that staff can call upon it in the immediacy of a threatening crisis, as well as in formal group or individual therapy sessions. All staff need to be equipped with the skills and knowledge to choose from a range of effective responses to challenging behaviour. Training in several models means that staff will have available a range of convincing alternatives to moral judgement and condemnation. In its application to the management of daily life on psychiatric wards, and the management of psychosocial crises such as imminent violence, the range of knowledge, understanding and skill required is as yet poorly codified. There are perhaps reservoirs where it may be found, for example, among skilled psychiatric nurses, or among the staff of therapeutic communities. This research and, for example, the work of Johnson and Hauser (2001) on de-escalation, shows the way forward in identifying those skills and applications so that they can be taught more effectively to new staff.

Herein lies another problem, more specifically for psychiatric nursing but also partly relevant to other disciplines. There exists little in the way of teaching material and textbooks about the care, treatment and management of PD patients. It is hoped that this book may contribute to what will become a growing body of material with a practical application that can be used in training. However, there is much to be learned from US colleagues in terms of manualized training as a way of quickly equipping a large workforce with necessary skills. The availability of pre-prepared training packs, with overheads, videos, learning tasks, etc., would ease the way towards progress.

It may also be possible to improve selection and recruitment to PD specific services. Given the difficulties presented by PD patients, it seems likely to be unwise to allocate staff to work in these specialist areas without expression of a wish to do so. Those with pre-existing negative attitudes will find them self-confirming, elicit more difficult patient behaviour, and influence other staff. It would therefore be better to selectively recruit those who wish to meet the challenge of PD care. Experience at Rampton Hospital, and in the new DSPD services, demonstrates that that challenge does itself attract staff who will rise to it, who are willing to exert themselves, learn new skills, and reflect upon their own beliefs and approaches. During the selection process, it may be possible to assess candidates on the degree to which they possess the psychiatric philosophy, moral commitments, cognitive-emotional self-management methods, technical mastery and teamwork skills, which seem to be necessary to accomplish positive working in these environments. Thus it may be possible to choose the best people for the job, and at the time of writing, further research by the author is exploring this possibility. Particularly important is the recruitment of psychiatrists and psychologists for such a service. Other disciplines look to these key professionals for leadership, and they can make a critical difference to the achievement of success. Of course, an ability to select is predicated upon the assumption that a range of candidates will be available. Unfortunately this is not always the case: compromises have had to be made in the past, and may have to be made in the future. However when choices are possible, there are now some criteria to assist in making them.

Once those staff are recruited, they require a careful induction to the management of PD patients. This applies to qualified professionals of all disciplines and especially to unqualified, and junior inexperienced workers. Of course all will require the generic induction to the organization that is provided to everyone. However, because they are so difficult, specific and extra challenges are involved in the care of PD patients. This demands an extra investment in the preparation of staff who will not necessarily know what to expect or how it should be dealt with. That induction should include classroom instruction about the practical management of PD patients and their behaviour, making up some of the deficits in the basic training of those recruited (or in the case of unqualified staff, providing this for the first time). That should be followed by a planned introduction to patients and the care environment, backed up by skilled workers' demonstration of the managing of difficult behaviour in practice, and support for the new workers in dealing with the early challenges presented to them by patients. Additional time should be made available for reflection under skilled guidance upon emotional responses to patients (and their past crimes). Moreover, the ward team needs to make sure that the right messages (i.e. not cynical ones) are conveyed about the treatment, structure and philosophy of the unit. Early investment at this stage seems likely to prevent major difficulties later (e.g. gross manipulation of naïve staff), and to lay the foundations for an overall positive attitude.

All workers, from whatever psychiatric profession, who are working with PD people of whatever level of severity, need two further sources of support in order to achieve and maintain positive attitudes. These are access to further training, and ongoing clinical supervision. Further training should specialize in PD care and treatment. Until recently such training was rare and hard to obtain in the UK, but it is now becoming more widely available. These courses enable professionals to spend time away from the clinical arena while they learn new skills, new ways of viewing PD behaviour, new treatments, and also provide the opportunity for them to exchange expertise, solidify team cohesion, and reflect upon beliefs and professional behaviour. The provision of these courses allow professionals to progress while being involved in PD care, gaining new qualifications and experience, and maintaining enthusiasm. Miller and Davenport (1996) demonstrated in a controlled study that an educational programme might help to change negative staff attitudes to PD patients. In the absence of courses, or possibly in addition, staff should be enabled to attend relevant national and international conferences. Of course all this would take a real financial investment, in part to pay for the education and in part to have enough staff to enable people to be released to engage in it. However, if satisfactory care environments are to be achieved, such investment is required.

The study reported here also demonstrates the strong link that couples regular clinical supervision and overall positive attitudes to PD. Indeed, clinical supervision can be the key to learning good lessons from the crucible of direct patient contact. Yet again, strong organizational support and investment are required to make this happen, and to encourage staff to engage in the process. Without that support and investment, the struggle to set up and continue one-to-one meetings with a supervisor can become exhausting for the individual staff member and, in the end, impossible to continue. As can be seen from this report, clinical supervision has become fairly well embedded in nursing practice. This does not seem to be the case for other psychiatric disciplines, most notably medical staff but possibly also psychologists. These disciplines are also likely to find the practice helpful, and should be assisted, encouraged and financed to find expert clinical supervisors from whom they can obtain regular support and development.

Extra effort also needs to be made by everyone involved in PD care to prevent the splitting that so easily occurs between points of tension. These comprise the natural divisions between different disciplines, and between staff and their managers. Because of the ways PD patients behave (and staff respond to them), particular attention needs to be paid to securing cohesion between different professional groups, which means allocating extra time to discussion, exchanges of views, mutual consultation and agreeing actions. In relation to management, the typical fracture point is that between the working team that deals face-to-face with PD patients, and those above. The working team tends to be cohesive in the face of the external threat from patients, however more senior managers are not incorporated in this sense of 'the team' because they are not exposed to the same threat. In order for managers to contain this point of tension, a management style (and structure) needs to be created where the immediate managers of the clinical teams have a real presence in the clinical areas, maintaining a first-hand knowledge of staff and patients. Ordinary management of the more distant, arm's length variety, simply does not seem to function well with PD care. The managers need to be present to express support and understanding, and to communicate and explain higher management decisions in a respectful way. The organization as a whole needs to achieve very high levels of clarity about (1) where the various decisions about patients are made, (2) who has responsibility for them, and (3) what latitude of action is allowed to staff in the front line. The staff on the front line (and their immediate leaders) need to commit themselves to this structure, creating their own appropriate ward rules and routine within it, consistently applying it to patients, and prepared to be overruled on occasion. Perhaps, in order to attain interpenetration of different levels of the hierarchy, front line workers could also have a high level of presence on management groups, as listeners, observers, advisers or commentators where an executive role would not be appropriate.

Some attention also needs to be given to the points of tension, jealousy and dispute between the different psychiatric professions. These are ubiquitous and problematic. For example, Jones (2002) describes a process which he calls 'professional degradation', in which the interventions of one's own profession are overvalued and those of others undervalued or considered to be of no importance. In work examining the operation of Community Mental Health Teams, Simpson (2002) eloquently describes how the stance taken by the consultant psychiatrist towards leadership of the multidisciplinary team can either facilitate or radically undermine morale and efficiency. These boundaries between professions form another weak point against which the splitting leverage of PD manipulation is targeted. Multidisciplinary teams therefore need to look after themselves, ensuring open communication, consistency towards patients, mutual support and mutual respect. Inter-professional education might be one route towards this goal; and further research on how some teams effectively accomplish unity might be another.

The organization as a whole can also help to facilitate positive attitudes by an open acknowledgement that PD care is highly challenging and difficult. This can be done by giving support and help to those who are victims of patient violence, making personal visits and expressing sympathy and encouragement. This might also be achieved by the securing of third party support for those undergoing the formal complaints procedure. The current procedure can be extremely psychologically damaging to staff and is sometimes abused by patients to exercise control over managers and staff. However, it must be acknowledged that, given the past history of the High Security Hospitals, it is difficult to see how things can be changed. Perhaps some form of remedy can be effected by making sure that support and help are given from elsewhere (managers cannot provide it as they are charged with carrying out the investigation), or by having the investigation completed by a third party to enable the managers to give support. At the very least, complaints should be dealt with rapidly so that staff do not spend long periods of uncertainty, suspended from their work. Finally, managers can acknowledge the difficulty of the job by providing a positive route out of the PD care arena for those staff who, by no fault of their own, are perhaps not suited to working with PD patients, or who are exhausted and burnt out from doing so.

The issue of the complaints process is a thorny one. In order to secure the balance between patients and staff, it may be necessary to retain it in its current form – in which case it might be better understood and accepted by staff if they appreciated their professional history and inheritance that have made it a necessity. Again, this is a recommendation that professional training should incorporate content on the public inquiries that have taken place into psychiatric care since the late 1960s, so that staff have the relevant background information to understand the action of their managers in the present.

To describe things in the above manner appears to load all the responsibility for achieving positive attitudes onto the organization and management. This is not intended, as individual professionals are also responsible for themselves, their education and their own attitudes. All psychiatric professionals working with PD patients may wish to reflect upon their own beliefs and attitudes in the light of the research reported here, just as the author has had cause to do many times in the course of analysing the data. Each of us is responsible for ensuring that, in terms of knowledge and skills, we secure adequate preparation for what we do and obtain effective clinical supervision. We need to consider the ways we work, how we perceive and interpret the behaviour of our PD patients, and how we morally evaluate both them and ourselves. Although there can be no final answers to these questions, the process of questioning ourselves is beneficial in its own right, and cannot but help to contribute to positive attitudes.

Application to general psychiatry

The lessons from this study are not restricted to forensic psychiatric services or PD specialist services. People suffering from PD are to be found in all branches of psychiatric services, from outpatient and community care through to inpatient acute care. The vast majority have never committed any crime, save perhaps minor or occasional misdemeanours. Yet their behaviour is problematic, often to themselves because of its consequences and the handicaps it produces, but more often to those around them. That behaviour arouses in professional staff feelings of anger, fear, pessimism and exhaustion. As a consequence, they are generally disliked, and are unpopular with all psychiatric disciplines at all times. As documented in the introduction to this study, that unpopularity can lead to withdrawal by staff, and, in inpatient settings, precipitate suicide attempts by patients.

People with a PD are sometimes admitted to acute psychiatric wards when their personal lives become unstable, they are distressed, and are possibly threatening suicide. While inpatients, they engage in nearly all the same behaviours as those described in this study. As such, they are disruptive of the care of others, cause arguments and disagreements between staff, and foment much disruption. In a sense, their behaviour is harder to contain and manage within the context of an open, unlocked, acute psychiatric ward, staffed by psychiatric professionals who have not been specifically prepared to work with this patient group. In consequence, regardless of their distress or potential danger to others, they tend to be admitted with reluctance and discharged with great alacrity. Most patients admitted to acute psychiatric care do not have a primary diagnosis of PD, but rather suffer from acute psychosis, most typically a relapse of schizophrenia. However, many are young men, admitted because while in a state of relapse they pose a potential danger to themselves or others, and many of these in addition meet the criteria for antisocial personality disorder (Bach-y-Rita *et al.* 1971). They, too, behave while inpatients in similar ways to PD patients, challenging the rules, absconding from the ward, refusing medication, and becoming involved in fights and arguments with staff and other patients (Bowers 2001). They, too, elicit some of the same emotional reactions from staff.

In these ways the findings of this study are equally applicable to inpatient general psychiatric settings. A clear structure, fairly applied by staff in a spirit of equality, integrity, honesty, with the courage to confront difficult behaviour, is needed in order to achieve a stable therapeutic environment. Staff need the right skills in team working and technical mastery in order to manage patient behaviour positively and therapeutically. The right attitude of staff, expressed through a containment of their own emotional reactions and an expression of their moral commitments, elicits less disturbed and manipulative behaviour from patients. When that behaviour does occur, positive attitude staff are able to transform it into a therapeutic learning opportunity. The means to achieve overall positive attitudes among staff will also be similar to those described in the preceding section.

This study highlights two false dichotomies in current debates about the care of inpatients. Those debates impact upon care in both forensic and general psychiatric settings, and are therefore best considered here. The first is the current version of the old dichotomy between psychodynamic and behavioural approaches. At the psychodynamic pole are those who argue for the necessity of understanding ourselves and others, and the relationships between us (staff) and them (patients), using the intellectual framework of defence mechanisms, etc. At the other pole are those arguing for education in the technical skills of cognitive-behavioural interventions and other evidenced-based (i.e. supported by randomized controlled clinical trials) modes of treatment. At the heart of this current dichotomy is the distinction drawn between relating to patients as human beings, and psychologically intervening with them as 'others'. The findings of the research show this to be a false division and that, in fact, to lay the basis for a positive overall attitude to PD, we need both an understanding of the relationships and what that may convey in terms of the meaning of patient behaviours, and the technical mastery to intervene appropriately and grasp opportunities for the provision of therapeutic learning.

The second false dichotomy is related to the first, and usually goes under the title of care vs. control. At one pole are those who prioritize and emphasize the therapeutic role of nurses and, at the other, those who focus on the necessity of providing security and control over disturbed people who cannot be fully responsible for themselves. This dichotomy can be seen in the debate over special observation (the allocation of a nurse to watch over a single disturbed patient), with the 'carers' arguing for the abolition of the procedure, and the 'controllers' arguing for its retention on the grounds of patient safety (Bowers 2001). Other research by Clarke (1996), who conducted participant observation on a Regional Secure Unit, suggested that psychiatric nurses fell into one camp or the other. The research reported here does not support that finding. Instead it was discovered that positive attitude nurses who were engaged with patients, interacting at high frequency, were just as concerned about the maintenance of order and control as were the other nurses. This is yet again another false dichotomy, another debate, in which the differing positions need to merge and the arguments to cease.

The rejecting attitudes of psychiatric professionals towards PD patients can carry over into community settings. Community staff (for example psychiatrists and community psychiatric nurses) are reluctant to accept referrals of PD people, often feeling that there is nothing they can do for them, and that they only cause endless crises and trouble. Yet this rejecting attitude is a function of their psychiatric philosophy, moral commitments, cognitive-emotional self-management mechanisms, etc., just as in the hospital environment. Even an effective structure can be attained in community management through careful agreement and consistency to a management plan by all those involved. To achieve this requires training and supervision in appropriate care and treatment for this patient group, just as it does in the High Secure Hospital environment.

Societal attitudes to PD

In conclusion, the work reported here also raises questions about the attitudes of society in general towards people who behave in ways that can be called personality disordered. What values and morals does our society uphold in dealing with these problematic individuals, and how do social structures aid or provide channels for individuals in handling their natural emotional reactions towards PD people? There are no clear answers to these questions, as the ways in which we, as a society, deal with the issue of PD are not consistent. However, this is under review in the UK, and likely to change substantively in the next few years.

At present, those with a PD who commit serious crimes may be treated as ordinary citizens and sentenced to a term of imprisonment, but a significant number of long-term prisoners meet the criteria for several PD diagnostic categories. The message conveyed is that PD is not recognized as a disorder of any kind, but is bad character and behaviour that must be primarily punished and contained. On the other hand, a smaller number of PD people who commit serious crimes are considered mentally disordered in some way, and sent to the High Security Psychiatric Hospitals under Mental Health legislation. This implies that PD is seen as a condition requiring treatment and containment. To complicate matters further, people with PD are sometimes transferred from prison to High Secure settings in order to undergo treatment.

Part of the problem here is that PD challenges our perception of the criminal act, and the moral discourse of judgement and punishment within which it is embedded. If the person with PD is to be seen as a warped, misunderstood misfit, made such by inheritance and upbringing, only partially responsible for his or her acts, then does this not hold for all crime? And if so, this implies that the justice system needs to be dismantled and replaced with an institutional arrangement based upon a philosophy of therapy and rehabilitation. These questions have no easy answers, as it is hard to see how the criminal justice system would then be able to express in any measured fashion people's need for justice and permit an expression of their anger towards the criminal perpetrator. Yet if society was to be organized around the values of the positive attitude staff, as has been described in this study, there would be a massive shift towards understanding and treating the PD criminal, even if there remained a punitive element to any sentencing.

There are indications that UK society is moving away from a negative perspective towards a positive view of PD patients as 'misunderstood misfits', with the setting up of new services for Dangerous and Severely Personality Disordered (DSPD) people. These services are currently being piloted in both prison and High Security Hospital settings. The intention is to provide a treatment and containment service that is neither solely medical nor custodial. Another example of a combined approach is to be found in the well-known TBS clinics of the Netherlands. PD people who commit serious crimes in the Netherlands have their sentence split into two parts, the proportion of which varies according to the decision of the presiding judge: one portion being a criminal sentence served in jail, and the second portion being a period of therapeutic treatment in a specialist TBS clinic.

One highly contentious element to the new DSPD service in the UK is the intention to preventively detain some people suffering from PD who are considered to pose a serious risk to others. This is being strongly opposed and contested by some professional organizations and civil liberty groups, and the final outcome is, at time of writing, unclear. It may also be seen as worrying that there has been an apparent move towards the courts convicting suspects of serious crimes on the basis of small quantities of circumstantial evidence plus a diagnosis of PD. It has been argued that this has occurred in the high public profile cases of Michael Stone (the *Guardian*, 15 February 2001), convicted in 1998 of a motiveless killing of a mother and her child, and Barry George (the *Guardian*, 3 July 2001), convicted of murdering a well-known television presenter. It would appear that UK society is becoming much less tolerant of the PD individual, and that social regulation and restriction of PD people is increasing. Some sociological observers may interpret this as yet another expansion of the 'psychiatric society' as defined and described by Castel *et al.* (1982).

It is, however, certainly also the case that there is investment in the expansion of services for PD people, partly perhaps because of greater debate and the impact of some of the high profile cases mentioned above. In addition, the introduction of more tightly regulated community care during the 1990s (e.g. Department of Health 1990, NHS Management Executive 1994a, 1994b) and a focus on the seriously mentally ill with complex social problems, has prevented psychiatry from continuing to keep PD individuals at arm's length from services due to their disruptive capacity. For whatever reason, there is more interest in PD than ever before, with more conference presentations, more publications, more specialist courses being initiated, and more specialist treatment centres being founded. Most notable among these expansions has been the creation of two offshoots from the famous Henderson Hospital therapeutic community, plus the investment in the DSPD services already described.

However, it seems to be the case that our society also expresses the attitudes of the negative staff described in this study. These are marked by extreme angry responses towards serious crimes, coupled with a refusal to make any concession for the perpetrator's past experience and upbringing. There is a desire to punish, punish and punish again those who threaten the public and make them feel vulnerable. In these ways our society embodies a negative attitude to PD, one in which society itself mirrors PD in its intolerance and vengeful actions. The ultimate endpoint, if these societal reactions became established, would be a wide-ranging use of the death penalty and other extreme punishments. It is startling that these attitudes are most stridently held and propounded by the least well-educated and prosperous sectors of our society (for example, the anti-paedophile campaign in Portsmouth in 2000, and the campaign in 2001 to increase the punishment of two well-known children – the Bulger killers – who murdered another child, reported in the *Guardian*, 9 August 2000 and 28 June 2001 respectively). These campaigning public movements arise in the very same social groups which themselves generate the majority of those who are PD. The lesson here, if there is one, is that the problem of PD screams out for a large-scale public health oriented preventative investment.

The combination of media interest, PD, and the public inquiry culture currently prevalent in the UK, makes for an intoxicating, and possibly on occasion toxic, brew. The combination can have striking, and occasionally diametrically opposed, outcomes. Many examples may be given. Such is the high public profile of some patients in the High Security Hospitals, that any attempt to be humane by hospital staff, to execute a rehabilitative programme, results in newspaper headlines condemning the psychiatric services for being too soft on criminals. On another occasion, as previously described in Chapter 2, an absconding paedophile PD patient made allegations to the press that resulted in a huge public inquiry lasting many months. The services were also blamed when a young PD girl, Sarah Lawson, was discharged from a mental health unit and killed shortly afterwards by her father, who claimed that he assisted her suicide – by holding a pillow over her head (the *Observer*, 20 May 2001). In this case, although the psychiatric services clearly explained that satisfactory care had been given, the fact that Sarah Lawson suffered from a PD and had a long history of self-mutilation and overdose attempts was relatively ignored by the press. They took the family's side, castigating the psychiatric services for failing a young woman suffering from depression. All this media attention makes staff tense, nervous, self-conscious and worried that whatever they do they can get nothing right.

Society as a whole seems to have a potentially unhealthy preoccupation with PD. The criminal justice system's willingness to convict partly on the basis of a PD diagnosis is coupled with powerful statements from trial judges, expounding on the evil of the crime and the criminal. These are then reported and expanded by the media, especially the popular press, providing readers with the ecstasy of revulsion and a cheap enhancement of their own moral self-esteem. All this occurs in the context of a society in which serious crimes committed by PD and pseudo-PD people are considered the most suitable and thrilling content for films and paperback novels, produced and sold in many thousands of copies every year. Quite what this says about us is unclear. It certainly says that we are frightened of and angry at the PD individual, two of the key aspects of a negative overall attitude to PD as identified by this study. Fear, because the psychopathic killer, as endlessly portrayed in the 'thriller' genre, is the distilled essence of everything we are afraid of in the criminal. Anger, because he or she always comes to a bad end, frequently dying nastily, much to our emotional satisfaction and celebration.

This societal context exerts a strong pressure on staff working with psychiatric services, a pressure in the direction of negative attitudes recounted by some of the interviewees in this research. Perhaps at best what this societal obsession with PD says is that we find PD people different in interesting ways, and are fascinated and intrigued, curious to know what makes them behave as they do. On learning about PD, and perhaps in reading this book, it would be an entirely natural response to identify those known to us, past and present, who might be PD or have exhibited PD behaviour patterns. Students in the psychiatric professions pick this up rapidly, and it becomes part of their social discourse and worldview. However, perhaps it is possible to go further than this. If we look into the murky depths of the mirror of PD, we may eventually see a shadowy reflection of ourselves, of how we may behave when under stress and pressure; or we may see the tendencies we hold towards PD traits and the motifs from the symphony of PD that are echoed in our own lives. In learning, we may also have the chance to learn about ourselves, and discover what we have in common with those incarcerated in the High Security Hospitals. Then, perhaps, we may be prepared, if only in part, to be merciful to ourselves and to others.

Bibliography

Adler, G. (1973) 'Hospital treatment of borderline patients', *American Journal of Psychiatry* 130: 32–5.

Aiken, F. and Sharp, F. (1997) 'Containment and exploration: group psychodynamic psychotherapy for PD patients in a secure setting', *Psychiatric Care* 4(2): 75–8.

American Psychiatric Association (1995) *Diagnostic and Statistical Manual of Mental Disorders* (4th edition – DSM-1V), International Version, American Psychiatric Association, Washington, DC.

Barton, R. (1959) *Institutional Neurosis*, Bristol: John Wright & Sons.

Bach-y-rita, G., Lion, J.R., Climent, C.E. and Ervin F. (1971) 'Episodic dyscontrol: a study of 130 patients', *American Journal of Psychiatry* 127: 1473–8.

Beck, A.T. and Freeman, A. (1990) *Cognitive Therapy of Personality Disorders*, New York: The Guilford Press.

Blom-Cooper, L., Brown, M., Dolan, R. and Murphy, E. (1992) *Report of the Committee of Inquiry into Complaints about Ashworth Hospital* (Vols 1 and 2), London: HMSO.

Bowers, L. (1989) 'The significance of primary nursing', *Journal of Advanced Nursing* 14: 13–19.

—— (1998) *The Social Nature of Mental Illness*, London: Routledge.

—— (ed.) (2001) *Special observation and engagement*, http: //www.city.ac.uk/barts/ psychiatric-nursing/threads/spec_obs_engage.htm

Bowers, L., Jarrett, M., Clark, N., Kiyimba, F. and McFarlane, L. (2000) 'Determinants of absconding by patients on acute psychiatric wards', *Journal of Advanced Nursing* 32(3): 644–9.

Bowles, N. and Young, C. (1999) 'An evaluative study of clinical supervision based on Proctor's three function interactive model', *Journal of Advanced Nursing* 30(4): 958–64.

Brett, T.R. (1992) 'The Woodstock Approach: one ward in Broadmoor Hospital for the treatment of personality disorder', *Criminal Behaviour and Mental Health* 2: 152–8.

Brodsky, B.S., Cloitre, M. and Dulit, R.A. (1995) 'Relationship of dissociation to self-mutilation and childhood abuse in borderline personality disorder', *American Journal of Psychiatry* 152: 1788–92.

Burrow, S. (1991) 'Special Hospitals – Therapy v. Custody', *Nursing Times* 87(39): 64–6.

—— 'Therapy v. Security: reconciling healing and damnation', in T. Mason and D. Mercer (eds) *Critical Perspectives in Forensic Care: Inside Out*, London: Macmillan Press.

Butterworth, T., Bishop, V. and Carson, J. (1996) 'First steps towards evaluating clinical supervision in nursing and health visiting: theory, policy and practice development. A review', *Journal of Clinical Nursing* 5(2): 127–32.

Castel, R., Castel, F. and Lovell, A. (1982) *The Psychiatric Society*, New York: Columbia University Press.

Clarke, L. (1996) 'Participant observation in a secure unit: care, conflict and control', *Nursing Times Research* 1(6): 431–41.

Cloninger, C.R. and Svrakic, D.M. (2000) 'Personality Disorders', in B.J. Sadock and V.A. Sadock (eds) *Kaplan and Sadock's Comprehensive Textbook of Psychiatry*, Vol. 2, Philadelphia, USA: Lippincott, Williams & Wilkins.

Cohen, H. and Filipczak, J. (1971) *A New Learning Environment*, San Francisco: Jossey-Bass.

Coid, J. (1992) 'DSM-III diagnosis in criminal psychopaths: a way forward', *Criminal Behaviour and Mental Health* 2: 78–9.

Colson, D.B., Allen, J.G., Coyne, L., Dexter, N., Jehl, N., Mayer, C.A. and Spohn, H. (1986) 'An anatomy of countertransference: staff reactions to difficult psychiatric hospital patients', *Hospital and Community Psychiatry* 37(9): 923–8.

Cremin, D., Lemmer, B. and Davison, S. (1995) 'The efficacy of a nursing challenge to patients: testing a new intervention to decrease self-harm behaviour in Severe Personality Disorder', *Journal of Psychiatric and Mental Health Nursing* 2(4): 237–46.

Cutcliffe, J.R. and Proctor, B. (1998) 'An alternative training approach to clinical supervision: 2', *British Journal of Nursing* 7(6): 345–50.

Dell, S. and Robertson, G. (1988) *Sentenced to Hospital: Offenders in Broadmoor*, Oxford: Oxford University Press.

Department of Health (1990) *The Care Programme Approach for People with a Mental Illness Referred to the Specialist Psychiatric Services*, HC(90)23/LASSL(90)11.

Department of Health and Social Security (1980) *Report of the Review of Rampton Hospital*, London: HMSO.

Dolan, B. and Coid, J. (1993) *Psychopathic and Antisocial Personality Disorders*, London: Gaskell.

Fallon, P., Bluglass, R., Edwards, B. and Daniels, G. (1999) *Report of the Committee of Inquiry into the Personality Disorder Unit, Ashworth Special Hospital*, London: The Stationery Office.

Farrington, D.P. (1991) 'Antisocial personality from childhod to adulthood', *The Psychologist* 4: 389–94.

Friedman, H. (1969) 'Some problems of inpatient management with borderline patients', *American Journal of Psychiatry* 126: 299–304.

Gallop, R., Lancee, W.J. and Garfinkle, P. (1989) 'How nursing staff respond to the label "Borderline Personality Disorder"', *Hospital and Community Psychiatry* 40: 815–19.

Ganong, L.H, Bzdek, V. and Manderino, M.A. (1987) 'Stereotyping by nurses and nursing students: A critical review of research', *Research in Nursing and Health* 10: 49–70.

Gunderson, J. (1984) *Borderline Personality Disorder*, Washington, DC: American Psychiatric Press.

Hamera, E. and O'Connell, K.A. (1981) 'Patient-centred variables in primary and team nursing', *Research in Nursing and Health* 4: 183–92.

Hawkins, P. and Shohet, R. (1989) *Supervision in the Helping Professions*, Milton Keynes: Open University Press.

Higgitt, A. and Fonagy, P. (1992) 'Psychotherapy in borderline and narcissistic personality disorder', *British Journal of Psychiatry* 161: 23–43.

Home Office and Department of Health (1999) *Managing Dangerous People with Severe Personality Disorder: Proposals for Policy Development*, London: Home Office and Department of Health.

Hughes, G. and Tennant, A. (1996) 'A training and development strategy for clinically based staff working with people diagnosed as having psychopathic disorders', *Psychiatric Care* 3(5): 194–9.

Hughes, R. and Morcom, C. (1998) 'Clinical supervision in a mental health in-patient area', *Nursing Times Research* 3(3): 226–35.

Johnson, M.E. and Hauser, P.M. (2001) 'The practices of expert psychiatric nurses: accompanying the patient to a calmer personal space', *Issues in Mental Health Nursing* 22: 651–68.

Jones, A. (2002) 'Unpublished PhD thesis; London: City University.

Jones, K. (1972) *A History of the Mental Health Services*, London: Routledge & Kegan Paul.

Kennard, D. (1998) *An Introduction to Therapeutic Communities*, London: Jessica Kingsley Publishers.

Kohut, H. (1977) *The Restoration of the Self*, New York: International Universities Press.

—— (1984) *How Does Analysis Cure?*, Chicago: University of Chicago Press.

Kullgren, G. (1985) 'Borderline personality disorder and psychiatric suicides: an analysis of eleven consecutive cases', *Nordisk Psykiatrisk Tidsskrift* 39(6): 479–84.

—— (1988) 'Factors associated with completed suicide in borderline personality disorder', *Journal of Nervous and Mental Disease* 176(1): 40–4.

Lewis, G. and Appleby, L. (1988) 'Personality disorder: the patients psychiatrists dislike', *British Journal of Psychiatry* 153: 44–9.

Linehan, M.M. (1993) *Cognitive Behavioural Treatment of Borderline Personality Disorder*, New York: The Guilford Press.

Livesley, W.J., Jackson, D.N. and Schroeder, M.L. (1992) 'Factorial structure of traits delineating personality disorders in clinical and general population samples', *Journal of Abnormal Psychology* 101: 432–40.

MacIlwaine, H. (1981) 'How nurses and neurotic patients view each other in general hospital psychiatric units', *Nursing Times* 77(27): 1158–60.

Main, T. (1946) 'The hospital as a therapeutic institution', *Bulletin of the Menninger Clinic* 10: 66–70.

Martin, J.P. (1984) *Hospitals in Trouble*, Oxford: Blackwell.

May, D. and Kelly, M. (1982) 'Chancers, pests and poor wee souls: problems of legitimation in psychiatric nursing', *Sociology of Health and Illness* 4(3): 279–301.

McCrea H. and Crute, V. (1991) 'Midwife/client relationships: midwives' perspectives', *Midwifery* 7: 183–92.

McKeown, O., Forshaw, D.M., McGauley, G., Fitzpatrick, J. and Roscoe, J. (1996a) 'Forensic addictive behaviours unit: a case study (Part I)', *Journal of Substance Misuse* 1(1): 27–31.

—— (1996b) 'Forensic addictive behaviours unit: a case study (Part II)', *Journal of Substance Misuse* 1(2): 97–103.

Melia, P., Moran, T. and Mason, T. (1999) 'Triumvirate nursing for PD patients: crossing the boundaries safely', *Journal of Psychiatric and Mental Health Nursing* 6: 15–20.

Mercer, D., Mason, T. and Richman, J. (1999) 'Good and evil in the crusade of care: social constructions of mental disorders', *Journal of Psychosocial Nursing* 37(9): 13–17.

Miller, S. and Davenport, N. (1996) 'Increasing staff knowledge of and improving attitudes towards patients with Borderline Personality Disorder', *Psychiatric Services* 47(5): 533–5.

Millon, T. and Davis, R.D. (1996) *Disorders of Personality, DSM-IV and Beyond*, New York: Wiley & Sons.

Moran, T. and Mason, T. (1996) 'Revisiting the nursing management of the psychopath', *Journal of Psychiatric and Mental Health Nursing* 3(3): 189–94.

Morgan, H.G. and Priest, P. (1984) 'Assessment of suicide risk in psychiatric in-patients', *British Journal of Psychiatry* 145: 467–8.

—— (1991) 'Suicidal and other unexpected deaths among psychiatric in-patients', *British Journal of Psychiatry* 158: 368–74.

Neilson, P (1991) 'Manipulative and splitting behaviours', *Nursing Standard* 6(8): 32–5.

NHS Management Executive (1994a) *Introduction of Supervision Registers for Mentally Ill People and their Continuing Care in the Community*, HSG(94)27.

—— (1994b) *Guidance on the Discharge of Mentally Disordered People from 1 April 1994*, HSG(94)5.

Noak, J. (1995) 'Care of people with psychopathic disorder', *Nursing Standard* 9(34): 30–2.

Paunonen, M. (1991) 'Changes initiated by a nursing supervision programme: an analysis based on log-linear models', *Journal of Advanced Nursing* 16: 982–6.

Plomin, R., DeFries, J. C., McClearn, G.E. and Rutter, M. (1997) *Behavioural Genetics*, New York: Freeman.

Podrasky, D.L. and Sexton, D.L. (1988) 'Nurses reactions to difficult patients, *Image. Journal of Nursing Scholarship* 20: 16–21.

Power, S. (1999) *Nursing Supervision: A Guide for Clinical Practice*, London: Sage.

Proctor, B. (1988) 'Supervision: a co-operative exercise in accountability', in M. Marken and M. Payne (eds) *Enabling and Ensuring Clinical Supervision in Practice* (2nd edition), Leicester: National Youth Bureau and Council for Education and Training in Youth and Community Work, pp. 21–34.

Rapoport, R.N. (1960) *Community as Doctor*, London: Tavistock.

Richman, J. (1998) 'The ceremonial and moral order of a ward for psychopaths', in T. Mason and D. Mercer (eds) *Critical Perspectives in Forensic Care: Inside Out*, London: Macmillan Press.

—— (1999) 'Talking of evil in a special hospital: vignette research', Paper presented to BSA Medical Sociology Conference, York.

Robins, L.N. (1966) *Deviant Children Grown Up: A Sociological and Psychiatric Study of Sociopathic Personality*, Baltimore: Williams & Wilkins.

Rosenbluth, M. (1991) 'New uses of countertransference for the inpatient treatment of borderline personality disorder', *Canadian Journal of Psychiatry* 36: 280–4.

Sellars, C. (1992) 'The use of the Luria Nebraska neuropsychological battery in the assessment of mentally abnormal offenders: a preliminary study as to the nature of impairment and its relation to admission rates', Unpublished paper, Broadmoor Hospital. Quoted in Dolan, B. and Coid, J. (1993) *Psychopathic and Antisocial Personality Disorder*, London: Gaskell.

Severinsson, E.I. and Hallberg, I.R. (1996) 'Systematic clinical supervision, working milieu and influence over duties: the psychiatric nurse's viewpoint – a pilot study', *International Journal of Nursing Studies* 33(4): 394–406.

Sheppard, D. (1996) *Learning the Lessons* (2nd edition), London: The Zito Trust.

Sidley, G. and Renton, J. (1996) 'General nurses' attitudes to patients who self-harm', *Nursing Standard* 10(30): 32–6.

Simpson, A. (2001) 'Unpublished PhD thesis, Brighton: Brighton University.

Smith, M.E. and Hart, G. (1994) 'Nurses' responses to patient anger: from disconnecting to connecting, *Journal of Advanced Nursing* 20: 643–51.

Special Hospitals Service Authority (1993) *Report of the Committee of Inquiry into the death in Broadmoor Hospital of Orville Blackwood and a Review of Two Other Afro-Caribbean Patients: Big Black and Dangerous*, London: SHSA.

Spitzer, R.L., Endicott, J. and Gibbon, M. (1979) 'Crossing the border into borderline personality and borderline schizophrenia. The development of criteria', *Archives of General Psychiatry* 36: 17–24.

Storey, L., Dale, C. and Martin, E. (1997) 'Social therapy: a developing model of care for people with personality disorder', *Nursing Times Research* 2(3): 210–19.

Suokas, J. and Lonnqvist, J. (1989) 'Work stress has negative effects on the attitudes of emergency personnel towards patients who attempt suicide', *Acta Psychiatrica Scandinavica*, 79: 474–80.

Tennant, A. and Hughes, G. (1997) 'Issues in nursing care for patients with severe personality disorder', *Mental Health Practice* 1(1): 10–16.

—— (1998) 'Men talking about dysfunctional masculinity: an innovative approach to working with aggressive, personality disordered offender-patients', *Psychiatric Care* 5(3): 92–9.

Tilt, R., Cormac, M., Maguire, N. and Preston, M. (2000) *Report of the Review of Security at the High Security Hospitals*, London: Department of Health.

Watts, D. and Morgan, G. (1994) 'Malignant alienation: danger for patients who are hard to like', *British Journal of Psychiatry* 164: 11–15.

Wilkin, P. (1988) 'Someone to watch over me', *Nursing Times* 84(33).

Wilkin, P., Bowers, L. and Monk, J. (1997) 'Clinical supervision: managing the resistance', *Nursing Times* 93(8): 48–9.

World Health Organization (1989) *International Classification of Diseases* (10th edition – ICD-10), Chapter V(F), Mental and Behavioural Disorders (including Disorders of Psychological Development), Geneva: WHO.

Yurkovich, E. (1989) 'Patient and nurse roles in the therapeutic community', *Perspectives in Psychiatric Care* 25(4): 18–22.

Index